High Praise for Privileged Presence

Providing health care to the sick and injured from earliest infancy to the end of life...or to the worried well, for that matter...is ultimately all about relieving anxiety. Accomplishing that privileged mission requires a partnership of equals between caregivers, patients and their families. The moving stories recorded in these pages offer memorable examples of success and failure. We owe a huge debt of gratitude to those who shared their experiences with the authors, and to the authors themselves for recording their reflections so faithfully. The indelible lessons that emerge should benefit every individual and institution involved in health care, now and in time to come. But most important of all, future patients and families will be the principal beneficiaries.

— *Richard B. Goldbloom OC, MD, FRCPC*
Professor of Pediatrics, Dalhousie University, Halifax, Nova Scotia

Privileged Presence provides a unique and valuable insight into the healing power of relationships and partnerships...whether among family or between patients and professionals. Told through elegantly simple and poignant stories, generously shared, this long overdue book is a must read for health care providers of any discipline at any stage of their career.

— *Terri L. Shelton, Ph.D.*
Professor of Psychology
Director, Center for Youth, Family and community Partnerships
University of North Carolina at Greensboro (UNCG)

How to hold all of what is written in this book without surrendering to the convenient outlet of cynicism? Instead, how to hold all of this and allow it to seep inside, under the skin, into the bones? Into the bones where it will turn itself into solidity, weight, the stability to meet the gravitational force of too much to do, too little time to do so, too many heart-numbing experiences that so often keep we healthcare professionals from turning toward and facing into the pain of being human? How do we learn to hold the rawness and tenderness, the vulnerability that is ultimately the source of our confidence and willingness to meet the people who seek our help, who count on our humanity as much as our technical expertise and more so, who hope and expect us to be humane and compassionate in the presence of their nakedness? Here is one way: Read this book. Let it break you open…Let it drop you below the first flinch and gasp of pain, below the conditioned stiffness, the old hurt and guilt, into that place deep within you that is capable of entering into and lingering for a time with the truth of these stories. It may save your life, open your heart, and feed your soul by offering you a way of meeting suffering with care, attention, and new found love.

— *Saki F. Santorelli, EdD, MA*
Executive Director, Center for Mindfulness in Medicine,
Health Care and Society Director, Stress Reduction Clinic
Assistant Professor of Medicine
University of Massachusetts Medical School

This book presents some extraordinary stories that are not only compelling reading but forceful in presenting viewpoints and messages that resonate with my practice experience, one that had its fair share of miracles as well as mistakes. Most of these stories brought home messages to which I could relate. Some were messages I wish I had received and understood far earlier in my education, training and practice career. [*Privileged Presence*] should be recommended to the attention of medical students and residents in training as well as colleagues in medicine as part of the lifelong learning in and for our profession.

— *Andrew Padmos, MD, FRCPC*
Chief Executive Officer,
The Royal College of Physicians and Surgeons of Canada

Privileged Presence

Personal Stories of Connections in Health Care

Liz Crocker
and
Bev Johnson

BULL PUBLISHING COMPANY
BOULDER, COLORADO

Privileged Presence: Personal Stories of Connection in Health Care
Liz Crocker and Bev Johnson

Copyright © 2006 Bull Publishing Company
All rights reserved. No portion of this book may be reproduced in any form or by any means without written permission of the publisher.

Bull Publishing Company
P.O. Box 1377
Boulder, CO 80306
Phone (800) 676-2855 / Fax (303) 545-6354
www.bullpub.com

ISBN-13: 978-0-923521-96-7
ISBN-10: 0-923521-96-8

Manufactured in the United States of America

Distributed in the United States by Independent Publishers Group, 814 N. Franklin Street, Chicago, IL 60610

Publisher: James Bull
Production: Dianne Nelson, Shadow Canyon Graphics
Cover Design: Lightbourne Images

Library of Congress Cataloging-in-Publication Data
Crocker, Liz.
    Privileged presence: personal stories of connections in health care / by Liz Crocker and Bev Johnson
    p. cm.
ISBN-13: 978-0-0923521-96-7
ISBN-10: 0-923521-96-8
1. Medical care—Anecdotes. I. Johnson, Beverly H. II. Title.

RA425.C855 2006
616—dc22   2006016990

CONTENTS

Contents

Contents

Contents

Contents

*We dedicate this book to our families
who have both grounded us and
provided the encouragement and
inspiration to work with others.*

ACKNOWLEDGMENTS

Privileged Presence has come into being because of the generosity of people's spirits, either through their encouragement, their thoughtful comments along the way, or their willingness to share personal stories. Many people suggested sources and contacts; others directly shared their memories, both positive and painful; and some offered constructive feedback and steady support.

On those rare, rare days when we questioned the value of this project, we had important "cheerleaders" who reminded us that so much in health care is positive, yet, at the same time, so much needs to be improved. Often, all we had to do was hear another story to be propelled forward.

The following people are all embedded in the heart and soul of *Privileged Presence*. To each and every one of you, we are grateful beyond words:

Marie Abraham, Susan Adair, Alex Aguzzi, Martine Andrews, Richard Antonelli, Hon. Monique Begin, Vicky Bennet, Holly Book, Janet Braunstein, Jane Buss, Carole Carpenter, The Kenneth B. Schwartz Center, Linda Clarke, Ellen Cohen, Maureen Connor, Jim Conway, Brian Crocker, Catherine Crocker, Suzy Crocker, Colette Deveau, Nancy DiVenere, Nancy Dugas, Susan Edgman-Leviton, Bertha Etter, Shannon Farough, Sean Farough, Wayne Fiander, Marlene Fondrick, Gerri Frager, Debbie Gillis, Stella Girard, Richard B. Goldbloom, Danny Graham, Geri Haight, Kathleen Hipwell, Lawrence Horwitz, Stanfield Johnson, Steven Johnson, Donna Koller, Betty Lacas, Judy Lavigniac, Ryan Liebenberg, Fay Lim-Lambie, Fiona Liston, Eve McDermott, Sandy McDougall, Kim McInnis, Scott McInnis,

Acknowledgments

Nancy Milford, Heather Mitchell, David Murphy, Sallie Patel, Ann-Marie Thomas, Kerol Rose, Julie Ann Rosen, Janet Ross, Michael Rowe, Kelly Roy, Anna Maria Rumble, Saki Santorelli, Juliette Schlucter, Bill Schwab, Terri L. Shelton, Harriet Shlossberg, Catherine Sloan, Bill Schwab, Terrell Smith, David Spero, Pam Stein, Deborah Stern, Donna Thompson, Ian Thompson, Sue Uteck, Debbie Yokoe, Katie Zedible.

Authors' proceeds from the sale of this book
are being given to the Institute for Family-Centered Care
in Bethesda, Maryland.

Introduction

WHAT IS PRIVILEGED PRESENCE?
WHY THIS BOOK?
WHAT MATTERS IN HEALTH CARE?
WHY STORIES?
WHY THESE STORIES?
WHO IS THIS BOOK FOR?

WHAT IS PRIVILEGED PRESENCE?

PRIVILEGED PRESENCE. One title, two words, three meanings.

Health care experiences are moments of "privileged presence." When people are dealing with illness or injury, their own or a loved one's, all their senses are intensified. Health care experiences are defining moments in people's lives, full of poignancy and power, and are remembered for years, often in vivid detail.

Health care professionals are *privileged* to be present with patients and families during these periods of heightened stress, which are characterized by courage, fear, uncertainty, and vulnerability.

When personal connections are made, then patients and families are also *privileged* to be in the presence of health care professionals, with their training, caring, and compassion.

And, last but not least, we have been *privileged* to be in the presence of those who were willing to open their hearts and share their personal stories for this collection.

Privileged Presence: Personal Stories of Connections in Health Care is a collection of more than fifty true stories about a wide range of health care experiences. At their core, the stories are all about people connecting with people or people missing the opportunity to connect.

The stories reflect different perspectives (patients, families, health care professionals), and a variety of health care situations and settings, from a seemingly ordinary and routine visit to a doctor's office to a highly charged and complex stay in intensive care. Some stories in this collection will disturb you; others will warm your heart.

You will see how the kindness of emergency personnel lifted a mother's spirits in a time of crisis; how a dismissive and arrogant professional undermined the confidence of an already vulnerable family; how a husband turned his sense of helplessness into a beautiful, caring way of providing support; how a parent struggled to make sense of her son's world of mental illness; how the many kindnesses experienced by a dying man motivated him to establish an organization to promote compassionate care; how two young parents were supported through the death of their first-born child and the birth of their second; how a hospital administrator dealt with the tragedy of medical error; and how an elderly patient was "released" by her doctor for asking questions.

WHY THIS BOOK?

THE IDEA BEHIND THIS BOOK IS SIMPLE AND HAS BEEN BREWING FOR SOME TIME. We have shared more than three decades of friendship and professional collaboration. In our different roles as teachers, nurses, trustees, health care advisors, and even simulated patients, we have seen phenomenal extremes in how health care professionals treat patients and families, and the degree to which patients and families are able to express their views, be heard, and be invited into a partnership of care.

In addition to our professional work, we have also had babies, raised children, cared for aging parents, supported friends, and cried openly in the face of tragedy and death. Our personal experiences on the receiving end of health care, directly and with family members and friends, have underscored our belief that the delivery of health care needs to be more patient- and family-centered.

We have travelled unique paths in our two countries but have both worked locally, nationally, and internationally for changes in health care. We have spoken to large audiences, consulted in boardrooms, brought together people with conflicting views to build consensus, written articles, and produced documentary films.

Over the years, we have shared many stories about health care with each other. We have often mused, "If only everyone could hear these stories! Surely, then, people would see how important it is to fully connect with each individual patient, not just their illness." We have asked ourselves questions like, "How can families become empowered and understand that they have a right to ask questions?" or "Why are some health care professionals compassionate while others appear to be indifferent?"

At the same time, people were often asking us questions like, "Where can I get a book that describes what I'm going through? Where can I read about the health care experiences of others? Where can I learn from those who have shown the courage to bring about change?"

These questions of our friends and colleagues built on our questions, and we finally asked ourselves, "Could a book of personal health care stories show the world what we have learned and care so much about? Could such a book be of value?" Our answer was to put together this collection.

One way to think of *Privileged Presence* is as a support group in a book. People want to know about others who have been there, who have gone down the same path, and who have some understanding about the experience.

The stories in *Privileged Presence* share the wisdom of personal experiences so that all readers can gain new insights. Some stories will provide the comfort of familiarity; some will inspire the confidence for patients to become actively engaged in their own health care; some will speak to the compassion of clinicians; some will evoke the courage and determination to make a change in a hospital practice or policy; and some will simply and quietly support intuition and instincts.

While each story in *Privileged Presence* is different, they all echo the importance of honoring the uniqueness of patients and families and acknowledging their concerns, worries, and values. The collection as a whole offers powerful messages about the essential ingredients of "good" health care: respect; compassion; collaboration; open and honest communication; family support and involvement; and flexibility and responsiveness to individuals and their needs.

WHAT MATTERS IN HEALTH CARE?

OVER THE MORE THAN THIRTY YEARS WE HAVE KNOWN EACH OTHER AND WORKED TOGETHER, we have become increasingly convinced that the common denominator in what makes a difference in health care is always people and how they communicate with and show respect for one another. We also believe:

♦ Patients and families have expertise, knowledge, and intuitive understanding about themselves.

♦ Health and illness affect not only individuals but also families, however an individual's family is defined.

♦ The patient is the most active participant in the healing process.

♦ Patients are more than a disease or injury.

♦ Honest communication and collaboration benefit everyone in health care partnerships

♦ Health care is rooted, first and foremost, in human relationships. Medical technology and technical expertise are only tools within those relationships.

Dr. David Leach, M.D., Executive Director of the Accreditation Council for Graduate Medical Education, when presenting an award related to fostering relationship-centered care, said that "all cooperative arts depend on relationship, and the number one problem in medicine today is finding a way to create the space where relationships can happen."

Clinical decision making must be rooted in human relationships. Medical equipment and clinical interventions, with all their advances to support diagnosis and treatment, should never replace or get in the way of genuinely listening to patients and families. Because medicine is an art as well as a science, relying only on medical science ignores the art of making human connections.

The desire for better connections in health care is neither frivolous nor inconsequential. There is a growing body of literature that reports improved outcomes for patients and families who are more informed, who participate actively in decisions about their health care, and who have practical and emotional support.

Many leaders in health care are reaching out to patients and families and inviting them to tell their stories and participate in everything from facility design planning to policy making. These connections and partnerships with patients and families are not just benefiting clinical encounters but are also enhancing the quality of care, ensuring patient safety, and improving patient satisfaction.

WHY STORIES?

WE ARE AN ORAL CULTURE. We naturally tell stories to one another. Stories are a way of sharing our lives. When we tell stories, we find out what makes us unique and what makes us similar, what connects us and what builds bridges away from a world of pain and isolation. We feel a special sense of privilege when someone shares a particularly heartfelt story with us.

Talk to anyone who has just been diagnosed with an illness, or a spouse who spent the night in the emergency room waiting for news, or a mother whose son who is learning to cope with diabetes, and you will instantly hear a story. They will describe encounters and anecdotes and how the people who cared for them and their loved ones made a difference in their lives, both good and bad.

Sometimes the recounting of an event can be cathartic. For example, the mother in the story "I Needed a Guide" told us that the telling of her story helped her see that she had actually "done some things right" in the immediate aftermath of this tragic event and helped her replace her feelings of guilt with a sense of competence.

Sometimes telling your story is a doorway to someone else's story. For example, the mother in "I Want My Children With Me" told us that she was able to share her story with her younger daughter. This created the catalyst for surfacing her daughter's recollections of the day that she'd kept to herself for a long time.

Sometimes stories are powerful tools for change. For example, when the wife in "Flying Blind in a Frightening World" ultimately told her story to her husband's physician, the doctor began to change how he relates to his other patients.

And sometimes stories are powerful tools for learning. For example, the administrator in "Learning From Tragedy" told us that the most significant changes made in his hospital have come from involving, listening to, and learning from patients and families.

Rachel Naomi Remen, author of *Kitchen Table Wisdom*, has said that "Facts bring us to knowledge, but stories lead to wisdom." Stories often bring us closer to our own buried wisdom and remind us of our courage. Telling stories and hearing stories reassure us that we are not alone, that we are part of a richly textured human tapestry of experience, that we are in wonderful company.

Stories can be powerful medicine. Sharing experiences and feelings through stories helps us make sense of our lives and process trauma and loss. In gathering stories for this collection, in interview after interview, people would say, "Every time I tell my story, I feel a bit better." Hearts opened. Suffering diminished.

WHY THESE STORIES?

THE PERSONAL STORIES WE'VE GATHERED IN THIS COLLECTION ARE BOTH INSPIRATIONAL AND INSTRUCTIVE. Some are simply heartwarming and show how connections in health care can be positive. Some offer clinicians new insights about the experience of care. Others give readers pictures of courage and role models for having the confidence to speak up and to demand to be included in decisions about their health care. Still others stimulate reactions of outrage, serving as illustrations of what needs to change in health care practices.

Readers will meet a nurse who delights in seeing her staff bring a husband and wife together; a father who wants health care professionals to remember all that his son could once do; a doctor who believes in the power of a hug; a young woman left alone in labor; a medical student who feels compelled to put his values in storage; and a woman with bowel cancer who has nothing but praise for those who cared for her.

Virtually everyone has at least one health care story. People were more than willing to share their stories, to applaud the importance of compassion, and to showcase the harm of insensitivity. All the stories in *Privileged Presence* are true, but many names have been changed to protect privacy.

How did we choose the stories? We looked for experiences that were simple but powerful, diverse but resonating with a ring of the familiar. The stories chosen for this book were selected as ones that illustrate a range of experiences.

Many stories are so complex that they demonstrate both positive and negative aspects of care. Hopefully all will serve as inspiration for either what needs to be changed or what is possible.

The perspective presented in each story is that of the storyteller. In any given situation, there are always many different points of view; these personal narratives offer the storyteller's reality.

The stories are presented simply; they are plain, straightforward storytelling. The objective is to show rather than tell, to describe rather than preach. It is our hope that this unique and powerful collection of stories will touch readers in a variety of ways. Gentle wisdom is the objective.

WHO IS THIS BOOK FOR?

INCREASINGLY, THE GENERAL PUBLIC IS EXPRESSING CONCERN ABOUT THE IMPERSONALITY AND COMPLEXITY OF HEALTH CARE. Patients and families want health care professionals to connect with them on a human and personal level and to be emotionally supportive.

Patients and families also comment that caregivers often don't provide either enough information or information they can understand; they want information so that they can make appropriate decisions about their health care. Additionally, people feel that the health care system is a nightmare to navigate and to understand; they feel they must have someone with them to protect and advocate for them.

Patients and families, as well as health care administrators, clinicians, educators, and policy makers, all want to know what they can do to bring about change. We hope this book will provide some answers.

This collection of health care stories shows what works and what does not, what people want and what they do not, and what adds to or takes away from people's sense of confidence and well-being in the context of health care experiences.

We hope this book will make a difference to individuals and families and how they see their roles in health care. We also hope it will touch the hearts and minds of the professionals who work in health care settings and help them see that when you become a health care professional, the responsibilities and opportunities to touch people's lives are extraordinary.

This book is for anyone and everyone who cares about the human condition and can relate to the world of health care. The stories are as equally relevant to all those who have had a health care experience as they are to those who want to see changes in the health care system.

The stories can be read in private and reflected upon alone. Or, they can be the focal points for group discussions, raising such questions as: "What would I/you have done?"; "What was done well?"; "What needs to be different?"; "How does this story relate to what we are doing in our clinics and hospitals and what can we learn from it?"

We believe that you will be touched by the truth and wisdom contained in these pages. We cannot presume to know what meanings readers will take from these stories or how the book as a whole will affect their lives. What we do know is that these stories have inspired us.

~

As Unique As Snowflakes:
Responding to Individuals

"I was surprised that people with the same disease
had such very different stories."
—*Rachel Naomi Remen*

"People in their most vulnerable states
still just want to be people."
—*Suzy Crocker*

~

Illness and injury can create feelings of enormous vulnerability. In these circumstances, patients and family members long for someone to help them make sense of their upside-down world and relate to them, one on one, person to person, seeing them for all they are . . . not just an illness or injury.

Health care professionals may have seen thousands of broken arms, respiratory infections, gastrointestinal problems, strokes . . . but for each person who walks into a doctor's office, a health care clinic, or a hospital, what they are experiencing is unique to them. Their pain is personal, their fears are their very own, their ordered lives are now disoriented.

No two people, situations, stories are the same. Each individual wants to be seen, heard, acknowledged, understood, and recognized as a whole person, with a name and with a life. Such recognition creates the foundation for respect and dignity which, in turn, are the pillars for a caring connection.

I AM NOT A PATELLA
AUNT MARY
RESPECT FOR DIGNITY
FRIENDS IN LOW PLACES
WHO WILL WALK THE DOG?
UNRIDDLING THE RIDDLE

I AM NOT A PATELLA

It was a Tuesday evening and a regular modern-dance class. I was sixteen. I did a big pivot (fouetté) with big momentum across the room, but my foot stuck on the special floor covering used for dancers while my body kept going. I heard a pop. My leg was at a funny angle, and one of the teachers straightened it, but my kneecap was still in the wrong place. The pain was excruciating.

The ambulance guys were nice, but I felt every pothole on the way to the hospital. I waited in emergency for a long time with ice on my leg but with nothing else to numb the pain. About six hours later, the verdict was in. My kneecap (called a patella) was on the side of my leg. Surgery would be needed to put it back in place, but there was too much swelling to operate right away. Surgery was scheduled for Thursday morning. In the meantime, my leg was wrapped in a padded splint. The hospital staff thought I'd be more comfortable waiting at home.

My mum and I wondered how I'd even get into the car, let alone into the house and up the stairs at home. But home we went at 3 A.M., via an all-night drugstore for crutches. It was freezing cold and snowing outside. When we pulled up to my house, we first talked our way through how this would work. I couldn't lower my leg without experiencing shards of pain in my leg and so while I would try to use the new crutches, my mum would hold my injured leg up at a right angle to my body. With ice on the pathway, it was going to be tricky. A poor, unsuspecting newspaper delivery man ended up helping us navigate from the car to the front door.

When Thursday came, I was excited about the surgery, because I wanted to have my knee put back the way it should be. Of course, I don't remember too much after surgery because I was groggy, but I do know it was exciting to get a TV and embarrassing to use the bedpan, and I knew my mum was staying in my room overnight. Apparently the nurses told her that was okay, but there were no cots. So she created a sleeping surface by lining up two footstools and a chair and brought a sleeping bag and pillow from home. (Ironically, on the last morning, after three nights, a new nurse came in when my mum was taking her "bed" apart and said, "Goodness! You could have had a cot, you know!" Go figure!)

The next morning, a doctor I'd never met before came into my room with a bunch of other people and said to his group, "So, this is the patella." I tried to respond with, "Yeah, I'm Suzy," but he didn't respond to me. Did he think I wasn't there? He never told me who he was and never spoke to me by name. He just spewed out medical jargon to the doctors with him. I felt like a science experiment.

Didn't he know I was desperate for more information about what had happened and what would happen to my body? He was supposed to be looking after me, but I did not feel comfortable with him. How can you feel comfortable with someone who doesn't look you in the eye, shake your hand, call you by name, and tell you who they are?

Next, a physical therapist came in. All orders and no sympathy. She told me to get out of bed. This was the first time in four days that I had lowered my leg below ninety degrees. I've always believed that if something is super painful, then it probably isn't good for you. My leg hurt a lot and I was scared. She offered no alternatives as to what I could do. She just left.

Fortunately I got a different therapist the next day who was nice. She asked how my leg felt and if I was nervous. She was so encouraging and told me to just take my time. She actually showed me what she wanted me to do and how to safely approach the movements. I felt comfortable with her. She seemed to understand that, at the end of the day, it's about two people in a room trying to solve the same problem together.

The nurses were pretty cool. They showed me some little tricks to make it easier to move my leg, and one of them, even though I was going to be discharged later in the day, washed my hair. I can't tell you how good that felt! People in their most vulnerable states still just want to be people.

Suzy recovered fully and went on to dance again.

AUNT MARY

MY AUNT MARY WAS A LIFE-LONG SPINSTER WHO ALWAYS LIVED INDE-
PENDENTLY. Even growing up, I knew she was a force to be reck-
oned with. Aunt Mary was right even when she was wrong. I
loved her, I respected her, and I was a little bit afraid of her. And
so when she called me to say, "I want to go to the hospital tomorrow," I paid attention. I don't know why I bothered suggesting a
closer hospital, because Aunt Mary was set on the hospital she
wanted. She was also specific about "tomorrow" because she was
working that day, looking after a ninety-year-old woman.

When I picked her up, I could see that Aunt Mary was jaun-
diced. After evaluation in the emergency department, it was clear
she wouldn't be going home. This would be Aunt Mary's first
time in the hospital. Because she had no frame of reference for
that world, she had some unusual conversations.

For example, one day she told me, "This place is so stupid.
Some doctor was saying I should have a face-lift. I told him I
didn't want one and to leave." I was eventually able to figure out
that "some doctor" had been a hematologist who had been suggesting that Aunt Mary have some "platelets." Somehow, all she
heard was "face-lift."

On another occasion, obviously a doctor was trying to find
out what Aunt Mary would like in terms of "do not resuscitate"
orders. The doctor must not have been clear enough for her to
conclude that he was talking about her. She reported, "This doctor was telling me all these awful stories about what they have to
do to people sometimes. It all seemed gloomy, and so I asked him
if he had a happy family. He said 'yes,' so I told him he should go
home and spend some time with them."

Aunt Mary

And then one day, a social worker called me to tell me, "Your aunt is very frustrating. She won't have any care." They hit a roadblock, and instead of trying to negotiate the barrier with her, they called me instead. I told them that if they were talking to me, they obviously hadn't talked to Aunt Mary. I couldn't and wouldn't speak for Aunt Mary. Rather, I suggested that, if they asked her some questions, they might discover that Aunt Mary rarely had an unclear thought, felt she'd had an exceptional eighty-seven years of life, and wasn't interested in any of the hospital's invasive procedures.

Aunt Mary never wanted to be in the hospital, but we promised her she would never be alone. She was always surrounded by Irish music and family and friends. Even when Aunt Mary slipped into a coma, there were still people with her.

Initially, the nurses had been resistant about our being there all the time, citing some rule. As soon as I pushed a bit, though, the nurses caved in and brought chairs for us. The staff talked about how atypical it was to have people there all the time, but they could see how comfortable Aunt Mary was. I felt so badly for all the other patients who spent their nights alone with the dark.

RESPECT FOR DIGNITY

MY MOTHER-IN-LAW IS EIGHTY-NINE AND SUFFERS FROM A LOT OF PAIN FROM ARTHRITIS. Fortunately, Edith found a family practitioner who truly honors her wishes and requests.

When Edith goes for her regular physical, she doesn't go in and immediately get undressed. The visit starts with a chat. Her doctor says, "I need to talk to you first to figure out what we might want to do today." He always talks at eye level with her.

When the issue of an annual mammogram came up recently, the doctor reminded Edith of this diagnostic procedure. She said, "I've lived too long as it is. I certainly don't want any more mammograms." He replied, "I understand. It is my duty to tell you about it, but I respect your choice not to do it."

∼

Edith experienced the same respect for her dignity when she went to our small community hospital for surgery on her wrist for carpal tunnel syndrome. When she arrived, the nurses noticed that Edith was quite crippled by arthritis. They said she could stay seated in her wheelchair and only asked her to take off her blouse and put on a hospital gown, which rested on the rest of her street clothes. (She didn't even have to take off her bra.)

The nurses took her right into the operating room in her wheelchair and brought her back out again in the same chair after surgery. She never had to get out of her street clothes! Noticing the puzzled look on my face, the nurses said, "Oh, we've checked the literature. There's nothing to worry about with street clothes for this small surgical procedure."

FRIENDS IN LOW PLACES

MY FIRST ENCOUNTER WITH PETER WAS PROMPTED BY A PHONE CALL ON THANKSGIVING DAY, 1994. My sister, brother-in-law, and I were just about to go for an early-morning walk when a patient called me on my cell phone to tell me that there was "a guy in bad shape in the old dry-cleaning building" and would I please go and help him.

At this point in time, I had been working as a nurse practitioner at the clinic of a local shelter on Cape Cod for about a year. I was the first full-time provider and the first to work during the day. Staffing up to that time had consisted of volunteer physicians and nurses two evenings per week. Daytime hours were for outreach and continuity of care. I spent my first year going out on the streets and seeking out places where the homeless congregated. This became the cornerstone of my practice, and that Thanksgiving Day phone call was testimony to the fact that my approach was working.

I proposed to my sister and brother-in-law that we walk to the dry-cleaning building. They conceded but wondered why we needed to do this on a holiday. "Thanksgiving Day?" I replied, "What better day to help out someone less fortunate!"

Thirty minutes later we were looking into the open door of the old dry-cleaning building. Mattresses, bedding, a myriad of sleeping bags, blankets, and empty liquor bottles were strewn about. The place was dark and smelled of urine and stale beer. I stepped in and began looking around. My relatives watched anxiously at the doorway.

At first it seemed that the building was empty, but then I heard someone moaning. I moved closer to the sound, and there, under a pile of blankets, was a man who looked to be in his seventies with long white hair and a full beard. "Hello," I said. He replied, "Who are you?" I told him my name and where I worked. He was not pleased and cursed as he attempted to stand. He was highly intoxicated and had obviously not bathed, changed his clothes, or shaved in a very long time.

It turned out that Peter was fifty-nine years old and had been living on the streets for several years. This initial encounter was the beginning of several years of engagement, trust building, and eventual medical management of a myriad of medical issues related to Peter's acute and chronic alcohol and substance abuse. These complications included: bilateral hearing loss; depression; post-traumatic stress disorder (PTSD); personality disorder; chronic alcoholic hepatitis; peripheral neuropathy; exposure resulting in frostbite, gangrene, and amputation of his right big toe, as well as other toe debridement; multiple bouts of pneumonia; pancreatitis; skin cancer; peptic ulcer disease; multiple trauma related to falls and assaults, with resultant degenerative lumbar-sacral disc disease and lumbar osteoarthritic changes; and foot drop.

Peter's gait was unsteady, and he soon fell back to the ground. He went to the hospital that day against his will. From that encounter on, however, we began a relationship as patient and provider that eventually turned into friendship. Our relationship was often difficult, as Peter had many issues regarding trust due to a very abusive childhood. But persistence and consistency in my work with him helped him to learn to trust me.

In reality, we had a lot in common. We both grew up in Boston, we both were Irish Catholic, and we both had had an alcoholic parent. The difference between us was, "There but for the grace of God . . . ."

Friends in Low Places

Giving Peter unconditional love allowed him to grow as a person. Peter had a great smile, a quick wit, and a kind heart when given the chance to express his humanity. Sober, he was able to demonstrate compassion toward others and would often bring in snacks and little gifts to the clinic staff.

Peter struggled with his addiction and at one point achieved eighteen months of sobriety while living in a halfway house. But the real success came in January 2000. After being arrested while intoxicated, Peter decided to go into treatment one more time, and he never drank again.

In 2001, Peter decided to move to Pennsylvania. A friend who was a minister had agreed to help him find housing. Peter would call me every few months or so. In September 2005, he called to tell me he had a new apartment. He was happy, still sober, and connected with a church. He inquired about my family and gave me his new phone number, promising to stay in touch.

In early November 2005, I received a call from the shelter stating that a Peter K. had been found dead in his apartment in Pennsylvania. The coroner's office wanted to know if we knew of any next of kin. Review of his medical records from the local hospital revealed that Peter had listed me as his next of kin. I am in the process of having him cremated, and his ashes will be shipped to me. Once I am in possession of his remains, I plan to have a service for him.

Many of his homeless brothers and sisters will join me, as we have so often done in the past, to pray for Peter, and we will scatter his ashes in the sea. While I feel sad for the life that might have been, I am confident that Peter did find hope and joy in the end.

As Unique As Snowflakes: Responding to Individuals

———————

The nurse practitioner in this story has worked for twelve years to bring healing to the homeless, the underserved, and those who have been left behind. Her outreach efforts have taken her on to the streets, inside derelict buildings, and into the woods. She says, "I have friends in very low places."

Over a number of years, her efforts expanded an intermittent, weekly, one-woman nursing service to a full-time multiservice medical-health clinic with twenty employees. This energetic and tireless woman explains that she eventually became burned out from dealing with bureaucracy and administrative tasks and so stepped down as clinical director.

"I need to be able to talk to people. Everyone has a story, and I love to listen and help people figure things out. I never suffer from 'compassion fatigue' as long as I can work directly with those in need."

She believes that simple acts of healing can occur with each concerned question, caring visit, and reassuring touch. She bemoans the fact that many nurses never get to give baths or back-rubs anymore. "That's when you hear what's really on people's minds and in their hearts."

WHO WILL WALK THE DOG?

ODD THINGS SOMETIMES CAME ACROSS MY DESK WHEN I WAS WORKING AS THE HOSPITAL'S LEGAL COUNSEL IN RISK MANAGEMENT. One of my favorites was the request about a dog.

The charge nurse from the general medicine unit came to see me to find out if there was any legal reason why a patient couldn't have her dog stay in the hospital with her. My "lawyer" response was, "Probably not, as long as we get the proper release forms signed," but because I had been a nurse before becoming a lawyer, I was curious about the clinical circumstances.

It was quite simple. A woman had been admitted who used a wheelchair. She wanted to have her "helper" dog with her.

Now, as nurses we often refer to what we call "the evil-twin response"—you know, the response you might want to give but you know is wrong—and you always hope that when you open your mouth, the "good twin" will be speaking. In this case, the "evil-twin response" would have been, "You don't need the dog. We're doing everything for you." But it was the "good twin" who showed up in my office that day.

The "good twin" knew that you have to take patients as you find them. In this case, the woman had no family or friends. Her dog was everything to her and maybe the only living being who loved her.

To make a long story short, the dog was admitted. The patient was set up in a private room, and the charge nurse hired a dog walker out of the unit's budget.

UNRIDDLING THE RIDDLE

OUR FIRSTBORN SON WAS BORN FIFTEEN YEARS AGO WITH DOWN'S SYN-
DROME. If we were upset about this, it was for less than forty-five
seconds. We both very quickly realized that this was an opportunity and a blessing for us. Our early years with our son proved
us right. But I remember saying, "I can deal with Down's syndrome. But I don't know how the parents of a child with autism
cope." Little did I know I would have the chance to find out.

Our son had extensive language and played on the same soc-
cer team as his younger brother. In developmental language, his
"global functioning" was 85 percent. But around his ninth birthday, we entered a nightmarish world. He started behaving
strangely. In a matter of three or four months, he lost all language, stopped eating or dressing himself, and no longer prompted for going to the bathroom. His global functioning deteriorated to 10 to 15 percent.

We had no idea what was going on. Was this a psychological
problem? Was it psychiatric in origin? Was it a developmental
phenomenon? We turned everywhere for ideas and answers.

We had just moved to a new city. This meant that our son's
doctors had not known him before, but we had video footage of
him before his behavior changed so dramatically. In it, our son
was talking and laughing and interacting. We used this video to
impress on specialists that there was a once-happy boy inside this
nonresponsive person.

A year after our son's functional slide backward, when he was
ten, he had surgery to address stomach problems he'd been having for some time. After this surgery, he dramatically improved
and experienced a steep rise out of his doldrums. He returned to

about 75 percent functioning in six weeks. Then, as quickly as he had returned, he went back down into his hole again. For the past five years, his highest functioning has been 25 percent.

We decided to move back home, to the city and the specialists who had worked with our son before his functioning deteriorated. We wanted to be close to people who would be as driven as we were to try to make him better. When you have known a child who has been healthy and functioning and who then mysteriously declines, it provides powerful motivation to work to get this child back.

It's a lesson in human nature to understand that medical professionals are far more tenacious and thoughtful when they have an emotional connection to the potential improvements they can bring about. Our son's principal specialist was completely aligned with us emotionally, even when she was hitting brick walls. Like us, she wouldn't give up.

Some specialists have given up, which is frustrating. It's as though they've run through their standard treatments and, if nothing has worked, they want to move on to another person. Where's their curiosity? Why don't they want to try to turn over new stones? I believe our son is a riddle that needs to be unriddled.

I worry that we are missing the boat entirely. I can't help but believe that the secret to this riddle lies somewhere in the body-mind connection, in the gut-brain connection. We have researched as much as we can through the Internet and are now trying to secure a referral to a specialist in Massachusetts.

We are in the middle of this battle right now. It forms the context of our lives. We are battle weary. Just talking about it is a challenge.

I lie beside my son and listen to his stomach making noises like the Fourth of July. One of the hardest things for me is thinking that our son has been in chronic, constant, and terrible pain for years. I saw it on his face this morning.

We have two other sons. They love their older brother dearly and have learned that "we are all beautiful in our own ways." They play with their brother, cuddle with him, and rub his back and his belly. When they pray at night, they pray for their brother and to become professional hockey players. They tell God that if He has to make a choice, they want Him to make their brother better.

What would I like to say to health care professionals if I had one hundred of them in a room?

♦ Make your best efforts to be present for your patients in every way. You can be buried by these things, but the more you are present in the moment rather than processing, the better the experience for the patient and family.

♦ Know that patients and families can sense whether you are fully engaged and listening.

♦ Listen carefully to what parents say about their children's symptoms. Parents have insights and know the subtleties of their kids that can help doctors figure out what to do.

Is our son autistic? I don't know, in part because he seems more socially engaged than is typical for autistic children. We're told that he has a "chronic disintegrative disorder."

The most important thing right now is to think outside the box and to let go of ordinary expectations. It is said that you can't get clarity unless you embrace the confusion. I worry that the last five or six years in this state have deeply patterned our son. I pray that we can unriddle this riddle before he becomes stuck.

~

When Life Is Threatened:
The Importance of Support

"Great opportunities to help others seldom come.
But small ones surround us every day."
—*Sally Koch*

"You can do no great things –
only small things with great love."
—*Mother Teresa*

"A terminal illness affects the whole family,
and the entire family needs support."
—*Sue Uleck*

~

Support in health care situations comes in the same ways it is offered in ordinary, day-to-day life—concerned questions, reassuring touches, sincere listening, shared information, gentle truth, encouraging words. Sometimes, people suffering from illness or injury know how to ask for support, but others can be intimidated by the system, overwhelmed by their situation, or mired in a sense of unworthiness. Especially for them, support must be offered.

Support matters. Who among us does not respond to kindness, to concern, to love? When illness or injury strikes, a literal or figurative hand to hold, a shoulder to cry on, a functioning mind are needed.
Without support, people fare less well, recover more slowly, and suffer the additional trauma of being ignored, dismissed, or abandoned.

DEATH-LIFE
FLYING BLIND IN A FRIGHTENING WORLD
LIVING THE OPPOSITES
THE JOURNEY OF THE GREEN ELEPHANT
I NEEDED A GUIDE
RISE & SHINE
A PROFOUNDLY ISOLATING EXPERIENCE
HIS NAME MEANS "RISE ABOVE THE STORM"

DEATH — LIFE

I sat in shock as the surgeon
Uttered the dreaded word
Cancer

He said other things—like "highly treatable"
All I could hear for the time was
Cancer

I sat there trying to take it in
Or block it out
Cancer

I imagined he was anxious to get it out
And me out of his office
Cancer

What now? Wander out of the hospital
Tears flowing unheeded
Cancer

The word echoes in my head
Over and over and over
Cancer

I feel the urge to stop strangers
And tell them
"I have Cancer"

When Life Is Threatened: The Importance of Support

I know my world will change
Never be exactly the same again
Cancer

What emotions are evoked by that word
Fear, sadness, grief, anger
All of the above

First overwhelming sadness
Then fear for my people
Then surrender

My guides gather round
To make themselves felt
And to comfort

I am filled with a sense
Of love and protection
Of knowing

A sense that this world is only temporary
That there is no death
Just going home

When my time comes—my guides will be there
Reaching out to embrace me
And welcome me home

June 2004

Death—Life

THE SHARING OF THIS POEM OCCURRED IN A COFFEE SHOP AT THE VERY BEGINNING OF THE INTERVIEW. Moments passed in silence, the reader slowly digesting how effectively the words have captured the shattering intensity of hearing the word "cancer." The poem's author, a professional woman of sixty-three years, then said, "Every person who came into my life, from the point of this diagnosis on, was an angel."

Stella had had surgery to remove what she thought had been a persistent hemorrhoid that had been causing her extreme pain for two years. She was thrilled with the surgery because she could finally sit comfortably. This was her primary thought as she went to see her surgeon for a follow-up appointment.

He looked uncomfortable and said, "I have a surprise for you. This was cancer and I didn't get it all." He immediately added, "But it is 90 percent curable."

The poem captures the early moments and days . . . on to the angels.

When I went through the double doors of the Cancer Care Clinic, I felt completely cared for in every way. I was welcomed, and my daughter was welcomed. I was given a journal to record details of my treatments. The journal also contained every possible phone number I might want as well as a twenty-four-hour number I could call for anything—anything at all.

The radiation oncologist sat with me and my daughter and answered every question I had. He spoke directly to me and also included her. He never looked at his watch. He covered everything—practical suggestions regarding what kind of underwear I would need and prescriptions for medications I might need. He even covered really embarrassing things. It was as though he and the staff there had thought of everything for you, because they didn't want you to have any unnecessary stress.

My biggest fear had been that I might have to deal with arrogant idiots and be vulnerable to them. The doctors and all the other staff were more than I could have hoped for—completely kind, personable, and interested in all of me.

I have nothing but praise for the Cancer Care Clinic. I never had to wait, and there was even a fast track for getting our blood taken at the blood lab. The clinic area was as attractive as it could be (given all the necessary special equipment), and there was also a place called the Sunshine Room. This looked like a living room, and there was always someone there to talk to you, to give a massage or reflexology treatment, to lend you a wig or scarf. This was a public clinic, but I felt like a valued customer at a fancy private clinic.

I am interested in alternative medicine, and when I asked about different options, the staff would say they didn't know about this or that but never were negative about my questions. When I brought in something a friend had recommended, the staff had a pharmacist look at it for me. He took the time to examine every ingredient to see if it would be compatible with what I was already taking.

I was really anxious about radiation. I thought it would be humiliating, thinking I'd have to have my legs somehow wrapped around my neck. The staff showed me that it would be much simpler and more dignified than I had thought. I had twenty-five treatments, and, on the day of the last treatment, I came out and all the technicians were lined up to hug me.

The clinic showed everyone so much kindness. They were completely committed to every aspect of the whole person. I felt totally looked after.

There were things I did for myself, too. For example, I filled my balcony with flowers. I did guided imagery and listened to tapes for relaxation and pain. I also listened to a forgiveness tape that I think has added ten years to my life. My family had a "Spoil Stella Day." And my own spiritual practice was important. My spirit guides offered me a lot of unconditional love and support, assuring me that I'd be okay either way. They told me that if I wanted to stay, I'd be fine, and if not, I'd be coming home to them.

Do I have any advice for others? I would say, be prepared to be patient, stay in the moment, and live one day at a time. That's all we ever have... just one day at a time. And it can be a good day or a bad day. We can decide.

———————

Stella still goes for checkups every three months. Stella and her husband Paul have recently bought a house that she feels is her way of saying "yes" to her future.

FLYING BLIND IN
A FRIGHTENING WORLD

IN THE 1930s, A BASEBALL PLAYER, NEW YORK YANKEES' FIRST BASE-MAN, LOU GEHRIG, WAS DIAGNOSED WITH AMYOTROPHIC LATERAL SCLE-ROSIS, OR ALS. This disease has come to be more commonly known as Lou Gehrig's disease ever since. In the late 1990s, a former Canadian Football League player, my husband, was diagnosed with this same disease.

ALS is a terrifying disease. It usually begins in the lower body and rises, wasting muscles as it moves, until moving, swallowing, speaking, and eventually breathing become impossible. A person with ALS knows all this because the mind is unaffected.

What was the worst of it? My list is so long, but near the top would be the specialist. He may have had a lot of degrees, but he didn't know how to help us, and he had the social skills of a newt! The higher in the medical food chain you go, the more mysterious doctors become. I discovered that just because they have lots of degrees doesn't mean they have any common sense.

In July 1996, my husband noticed that one of his hands had started shaking. Our family doctor didn't think this was anything to worry about at first. My husband, from his days playing professional football, had a number of crushed vertebrae in his neck, and it was assumed that the shaking was a residual effect of the damage to his neck. As the months passed, though, there were other troubling changes. I can still remember the day we had a huge fight about tying his tie. He had had to ask for help and didn't like what I was doing—not a happy scene!

I remember going to the specialist with my husband in January 1997. He had had a number of tests for Parkinson's disease, Hodgkin's disease, multiple sclerosis, lupus, and ALS. The doctor said, "Your arm is not presenting the way I want, but I can't find anything specific." Funny thing is that I remember glancing through a pamphlet for ALS that day, in the waiting room. I thought it was the most depressing thing I'd ever read. Nothing clicked in about the symptoms it described.

On March 25, two months later, the specialist called us back in. He said, "I know I told you back in January that I couldn't find anything. Well, I was wrong." He went on to say: "You should quit your job; you need to convert your house or move; you have less than two years; there's not really a regime of drugs that will help, because this is terminal." All the while he was talking, he never looked at me. Who did he think was going to look after this man?

His parting words were, "I can see this is a lot to take in. I'll call you in a couple of days." He never called. From that point on, we were flying blind in a frightening world. The doctor didn't even give us that horrible pamphlet.

We would see this doctor twice a year. My husband, fighting so hard to continue to work, to be useful, to participate in activities with family and friends, would look forward to these visits. He wanted his efforts to be recognized. All the doctor needed to say was something like, "Gosh, you're hanging in there so well—good for you." Instead, all he said was, "You're about where I expected you to be." And, as always, he never talked to me.

How could he say, "You're where I expected you to be?" He had told us my husband would be dead in two years. In fact, he lived for almost six years, was only sick twice, and only missed one week of work in all that time. He worked until a Monday and died on a Wednesday. Imagine, "You're about where I expected you to be!" He had no idea what we were going through.

When Life Is Threatened: The Importance of Support

The only time this specialist ever acknowledged me on our twice yearly visits was when he could no longer understand what my husband was saying. He turned to me to ask me to interpret. I couldn't resist what I did. I'd been leafing through a magazine, listening carefully to everything that was being said but in the posture of one who is being ignored. When the doctor spoke to me, I looked up with the look of someone who has been disturbed from a good read and said, "Oh, sorry, were you speaking to me?"

As we scanned our universe for anything that could help us, we found a group at the local rehab hospital. This was great for a while, because they had a program in the pool to help reduce the stiffness in my husband's joints. Unfortunately, everyone else in the group died, and so the program was discontinued. I guess the fact that my husband was still alive didn't constitute a group!

We found the most useful information through the Internet, where we found an ALS group and could talk to both caregivers and patients from around the world. For example, when my husband started to choke, people on-line told us he needed a feeding tube. No one had suggested that we could be proactive. I still recall the day my husband sent me an e-mail saying he was losing sensation in his tongue. This was a man who loved food. The move to the feeding tube was huge.

One of the best tips I got from this group was to use a condom as a urinary leg bag. As my husband became incontinent, he was involuntarily wetting his pants. Without the tip about the condom, we would have had to use diapers right away.

I also learned some tricks for moving my husband. No one had told me how to lift him into his wheelchair or onto the toilet or a shower bench. I used to joke that I was training for the Olympics in the Clean, Snatch, and Jerk events.

This group was not only informative but also very supportive. I found out I wasn't the only person who dropped her husband on the floor. In fact, I could even share some tips from my
own experience. For example, one night, when I tried to get my
husband out of his chair without taking his socks off first, his feet
just slid across the floor, and we both slowly went down.
Everyone heard that one and the significance of socks!

The other great tip I got was that antidepressants help dry
up saliva. My family doctor got a prescription for us that was
such a help. Because my husband's tongue and throat muscles
weren't working any longer to swallow saliva, he had been
drooling constantly.

We had to go to the emergency room a couple of times. I've
never seen such an overworked and compassionate group in my
life as the staff in emergency! They always asked how I was
doing, which was more than the specialist did!

The only other person who asked about me was my family
doctor. She was fabulous, not just because she showed concern
for me, but because she'd get things for us and would follow up
on things that had fallen through the cracks. She would also
sometimes just call us at home to see how we were doing.

By comparison, our regular appointments with the specialist
were useless. We would ask questions about new drugs or treatments we had heard about, but all the doctor would say was,
"You seem more versed than me on this one." We were always
ahead of anything the formal system offered us. He never visited
us and didn't even come to see my husband when he had to go
to the hospital.

Do I sound like I was an angry caregiver? Well, I was. My
husband knew this and didn't mind. He called me the "family
ventilation system." I guess I would blow off steam for everyone.

When Life Is Threatened: The Importance of Support

For the most part, I felt I was on my own. We had great friends, some of whom cooked for us, or made the kids Christmas cookies so that they'd feel just like other kids when they took their lunches to school, and many of whom would come and sit with my husband and watch TV with him. But that just meant I could drive the kids to hockey games or music lessons or cook dinner. I needed a break, too. I was trying to be the family glue, maintain the semblance of ordinary life for everyone, and still go to work myself.

A regular day for me would involve getting up early to get my husband ready for work and the kids ready for school. Then I'd take my husband to work, go to work myself, pick up my husband for lunch and get him back to work again, go back to work myself, go back to get my husband, and be home for the kids after school. Then there were all the things that normally happen in a home with young children—homework, activities, a meal, bedtime—and then getting my husband ready for bed.

And nighttime was no picnic. I would have given almost anything for a full night's sleep. My husband described it best when he said, "On a good night, I only wake my wife up eight to ten times. On a bad night, it's every five minutes!"

I often wondered, "How long can I do this?" I felt so alone at night. When I was in the thick of things, I didn't have time to think. The feelings of isolation and exhaustion would come in the middle of the night.

Sometimes, I'd just go into the bathroom and sit on the floor and have a good cry. But I could only take a couple of minutes and then I was back in action.

How did I look after myself? I didn't! I existed on pure adrenalin. I put on thirty-five pounds and remember thinking, "How did that happen? I didn't even have time to eat!"

Flying Blind in a Frightening World

Did I have any heroes? Friends, my family doctor, the staff in emergency, and two nurses stand out. The encounters were brief but brilliant!

In the first instance, in the fall of 2001, we made a heroic effort to travel up to Toronto for the Vanier Cup, which is the biggest football game of the year in the world of university football. When we got there, my husband's feeding tube was clogged. We mobilized, making a call to the city's special taxi service and heading to a downtown hospital. Once there, we heard, "Oh, we can't get to that until tomorrow—he'll have to stay overnight." I couldn't believe my ears . . . all this way to sit in a hospital? An older nurse overheard what was going on and said, "Does anyone have fifty cents? Go buy a can of Coke!" Ten minutes later, the Coke had cleared the feeding tube and we were on our way. My husband's team won and the players presented him with the trophy.

The second nurse worked on an inpatient unit. It was one of the two times my husband actually had to be in the hospital during the five and a half years. He was in a four-bed room. The patient who had been in bed #3 died and the resident doctor wanted my husband moved to bed #3, maybe because it was a bit nearer the door. I overheard this nurse, outside the door to our room, take on the doctor and say, "No he's not going to bed #3. He knows someone just died in that bed, and he might think that's the 'dying bed.' He's going to stay where he is. A new patient can go to bed #3." The doctor started to challenge her, but she just cut him off, saying, "Listen, you young pup. You can write me up if you like, but he is not going to bed #3." Bravo! She deserved an Academy Award for Best Performance in a Supporting Role!

My kids? They were four and six when my husband got sick. They missed out on a lot—not only their dad, but time I couldn't spend with them. In a way, my kids are only now meeting the real me. My son, now fourteen, jokes with his friends, saying, "Great! I hit my teenage years, and my mom has time for me!"

My son and I have been in therapy for the last year. He had a lot of anger that I didn't tell him his father was sick and was going to die. We got his diagnosis in March and just wanted a couple of months to digest the information and figure out how we were going to go forward with all this. But the press got hold of the story. Because my husband had a high profile in the community, it became headline news without our knowing first. Some kid came up to my son at school and said, "I'm sorry your dad is going to die." My husband's father found out on a bus when he saw it in the newspaper. What was news for the media turned out to be agony for us.

My daughter seems to be okay. She doesn't really remember a time when her dad wasn't sick. His changes over the five and a half years were gradual, and she seemed to adjust on a day-by-day basis.

What would I like to tell doctors? I want them to know that a terminal illness affects the entire family. And that the entire family needs support.

Two years after my husband's death, I made an appointment to see the specialist who followed his case. I was in his office for an hour and just unloaded. I wanted him to know that he had ignored me and what that had felt like; that he had offered us virtually nothing at a time when we needed some sort of support and survival guide along with referrals to relevant resources; that he had no idea what we had to deal with on a day-to-day level; that the system had left us to fly blind; that it wasn't enough for a doctor to be smart—that social skills matter too. I wanted him to know that seeing a doctor every six months wasn't often enough—the changes with ALS are too dramatic and too fast for that. We needed to know that someone was on our team figuring out the plays before we got tackled. I told him that we had discovered the on-line group on our own—couldn't he have told us about that?

I described our experience of being seen in a clinic in another city in which all the relevant specialists saw the patients with ALS and came up with coordinated suggestions from various care specialties. I explained that while the patients were being seen, the family members got to meet together and find out what others were doing to manage, to cope. I added that, while at this clinic, we were given a book called the *ABCs of ALS*. I asked him why couldn't there be something like that here, especially given that we had the highest per-capita incidence of ALS and multiple sclerosis for the whole country.

Did this meeting make me feel better? Yes, especially when I started to hear from others in our community who had ALS and were served by the same specialist. Apparently, this doctor has changed and is now paying attention and relating to people in ways that feel very human. This is a good beginning.

LIVING THE OPPOSITES

JANE IS BRIGHT, ARTICULATE, FUNNY, ACTIVE, AND STRONG. At age fifty-five, she swims fifty laps every weekday, walks ten kilometers every weekend, and runs a large arts organization with a passion that is infectious. Jane's strength is not only physical (she has been known to crack ribs with her enthusiastic hugs) but also psychological (she can handle a lot of tough stuff). Jane was diagnosed with multiple sclerosis twenty-four years ago, breast cancer five years ago, and a troubling heart condition two years ago.

Jane points to a sign over her desk. It says "No Sniveling." "That's my approach to most things," she says. "I don't feel sick and I'm not into being sick. It's tedious, boring, and slows you down. I have no pain, no shortness of breath, no fatigue. I do have hot flashes from tamoxifen, but so what? That's no big deal."

Five years ago, Jane had not been feeling well, had found a lump in her breast, and had gone through a series of tests. At 4 P.M. on Christmas Eve, she received the news that she had breast cancer. A mastectomy revealed that twenty of twenty-four lymph nodes examined also were affected. She was referred to the Cancer Care Clinic to learn about her treatment options and was encouraged to bring someone with her to the consultation. Jane took a friend. She tells her story this way:

> Every step along the way, people were kindness personified. At that first consultation, I was scheduled for half an hour, but the doctor spent two and a half hours with us. He outlined a number of options, drew pictures, showed us graphs, explained procedures, and then said, "Now I'm going to leave you for half an hour so the two

of you can talk without me here. When I come back, I'd like you to tell me what your preliminary decision is for which option you want to follow. It's only preliminary, because you can change your mind during the coming week, but it will help us all start to focus on what's best for you." Brilliant! He gave us clear information, then space and time alone, all with no pressure.

I have nothing but praise for the Cancer Care Clinic. I could call night or day. The nurses were angels. I went through radiation and chemotherapy. It was positive, positive, positive. I felt blessed. But then I entered an entirely different world.

Because I am taking tamoxifen and a possible side effect can be cancer of the cervix, I promised to have regular Pap smears. But you know how life is—you get busy, you feel healthy, you forget. Three years into taking tamoxifen, I finally booked an appointment through my family doctor. I was a bit surprised that even though I called for an appointment in November, I couldn't get an appointment until January. Surprise turned to concern when the appointment was rebooked three times. But concern turned to irritation when I showed up for my appointment at 7 A.M. and waited until 8:30, and still my doctor had not arrived. That's when I left and turned my irritation into action into getting a new family doctor.

My new doctor, a tiny, wee woman who looked like a kid, was fabulous. I had my first full visit with her in early March 2004. In addition to doing the Pap test, she listened to my heart and lungs and took my blood pressure. "How long have you had a heart murmur?" she asked. "And how long have you had high blood pressure?" My blood pressure was 170/128. This was news to me because my previous doctor had never taken it. She never told me about any heart murmur either. It was Friday.

This new doctor scheduled me for an electrocardiogram (ECG) on Monday. The technicians repeated the ECG three times, telling me that they thought their machines were broken. Then they asked me to wait while they faxed the results to my doctor. She called me while I was still in the ECG room and said, "The ECG says you're having a heart attack, and I want you to go to the emergency room right away."

When I arrived in emergency, I discovered that if you have my kind of ECG slip, you get seen right away and get hooked up to lots of machines. The doctors and nurses were all shaking their heads as they looked at the jagged lines on the machines and asked, sounding skeptical, "You really swim fifty laps every day?"

The emergency doctors said I should get more tests. But four months passed and I heard nothing. Didn't bother me, really, because I had no symptoms, but I called my new family doctor to tell her that nothing had been scheduled. She made a couple of calls. Tests were scheduled.

What I remember most about that series of tests is that when I was on the treadmill, I never got tired. And yet, the technicians said things like, "Oh my god, can you feel that? Your heart is doing funny things." I found their comments somewhat alarming, but I didn't feel anything.

Living the Opposites

Next, I had a twenty-four-hour heart-monitor test. I was told it would take three weeks to get the results. After four weeks, I called. A receptionist told me I wouldn't hear for another two months. And that's when I started to make calls, leaving messages for the cardiologist, trying to sound like a squeaky wheel, or a dying duck, or a pathetic version of Swan Lake. Turns out, the results of the twenty-four-hour trace had been lost and I would have to repeat the test.

I got a message on Friday to show up for the test on Monday at 9 A.M. On Monday, I sat there until noon. I asked the nurse, "Is the doctor here, ill, or somewhere else?" She said, "I'll page him," and then left for lunch.

The doctor showed up at 1:15. I'd never met him before, but his first words were, "How are you, dear?" I started to get mad, but then I laughed. It was all so ridiculous! I explained that I'd had all sorts of tests because there was something about my heart that seemed to be alarming to doctors. This all had started in March and it was now September and I really had no idea what was going on.

This doctor was ultimately able to tell me what was wrong structurally with my heart (ventricular tachycardia) and suggested that I have a catheterization to find the specific locus of the problem. Seemed like a plan.

In mid-October, I went into the hospital on a Wednesday night to be monitored for thirty-six hours. The procedure was going to be on Friday morning. I was sharing the room with a woman who was very sick and in a lot of pain. It can't have been any fun for her, because

I kept setting the monitors off at the nursing station and the nurses would run in every twenty minutes to see if I was okay.

My cardiologist had said he'd be in on Friday morning at 7 A.M. to go over everything with me. By 8:30, a group of doctors (without mine, though) came in on rounds. My case was clearly interesting to them because it was so bizarre, but they talked among themselves as though I wasn't there. One doctor in the group was very opposed to the procedure I was about to have, believing it to be dangerous and clinically inappropriate.

While I appreciate that it's important for doctors to give patients a full spectrum of information about treatment options, having a disagreement in front of me, without involving me, is just not acceptable. You already feel very vulnerable when you're ill. The doctors' argument was extremely frightening and I just lost it. I started shouting at them, screaming, and then I burst into tears. My roommate applauded as the doctors scurried out of my room.

My doctor finally showed up and calmed me down. But by then it was too late to do the procedure and it had to be rebooked for two weeks later. And I'm supposed to be avoiding stress!

Then it was early November, and I was actually in the operating room, prepped and waiting for surgery. It was determined that there was still one more consent form I had to sign. And, believe it or not, the same guy who had been so opposed to the procedure two weeks before was the one who brought me the papers, and he was still trying to persuade me not to go ahead! I told him to "just scram and stop messing with my head." I had more important things to focus my energy on at the moment.

I was awake for the whole procedure. It normally takes two to three hours; mine lasted for more than eight hours. But it seemed to work, and the pictures they took the next morning looked like a normal heart. The doctors said they'd follow up with me in January. In April, I called them.

Two weeks later, I did the halter monitor thing, and ten days after that, on a Friday afternoon, I reported in to get the results. Another hour and a half wait and a new doctor came in saying, "What are you here for?" I told him I was tired of people not knowing who I was or what was going on. We ended up looking through the file together and found the test results. My heart was again behaving as it had before the surgery. I had to have another stress test.

I've now had that test, and, once again, I haven't heard the results. I'm still hanging and I don't like hanging. I'm not easily frightened and I'm not afraid to die. But this current situation—the not knowing—is stressful and I don't need it! I have a life to live.

I know doctors are busy and I try to cut them some slack, but I have a life, too. The doctors may not think I am as important as they are, but my view is that everyone is equally important. And I'm especially important to me. I just want to be treated as a thinking human being who has a full and complex life.

When Life Is Threatened: The Importance of Support

As a cancer patient and as a cardiology patient, I feel I've been on different planets. But this means I know what's possible. I've experienced how it can be. I've lived the opposites.

THE JOURNEY OF THE GREEN ELEPHANT

The coffee cup rests on a side table. On closer examination,
the table is, in fact, an elegant green porcelain elephant.
The woman opposite notices my gaze, sinks back
into a comfortable, stuffed armchair, and travels
back in time. She begins speaking.

Great Care and Great Love

IT TOOK ME A YEAR TO PICK UP THAT ELEPHANT AND BRING HIM HOME.
It's a long story.

I was twenty-eight, in New York on a business trip, and had
bought a beautiful, thigh-high, green ceramic elephant at an art
gallery the day before. I remember calling my mother and saying,
"I feel like I'm on top of the world. I have just picked out a wonderful, new piece of art, and I love my job and I feel great!" At
the time, I was unmarried and working in Toronto as a lawyer.

The next day I had a terrible attack of pain while walking
down Madison Avenue. I staggered into some little restaurant,
draped myself over a table, and waited for the pain to subside.
When I came home, I experienced a similar attack but this time
had to go to the bathroom. When I looked in the toilet bowl, I
gasped as my stools were bright, emerald green. I went to my
doctor right away. She gave me a stool test kit and said to return
with the testing complete. I never made it back.

By early the next morning, pain was gripping my neck, chest,
and side. I also felt like I was choking. A friend drove me to the

hospital and I remember urging him to go through the red lights. I knew I had to get help right away. I collapsed in the entrance to emergency. I heard someone yelling, "No BP. No pulse."

The next thing I remember is being on a stretcher that was being pushed very quickly down a hallway. A doctor, running alongside of me, said, "We're taking you into surgery. You're bleeding inside." I could see bags and bags of blood on some kind of dress rack near me. It was the beginning of the AIDS scare. I looked hazily at him and said, "I'm going to get AIDS!" He replied, "Lady, that's the least of your concerns."

I heard that the doctor got into trouble for what he said, but I think he saved my life. There was something about his intensity and seriousness that made me click into survival mode. My mind whispered, "Pamela—participate!" This I did as much as I could from then on. I knew I had to participate to live, to keep my soul in my body.

I was on the operating table for more than fifteen hours. It turned out I had a hepatic adenoma, which is a single-cell, benign tumor. It had exploded and blown my liver and gall bladder into pieces. Following the resection of my liver, apparently I kept bleeding out. While the team of surgeons tried to stabilize me, a determined hematologist kept trying to mix potions for me in his lab. He wouldn't quit. Thank heaven!

Of course, I was only told about the medical facts of this very long day much later. Some of the details I heard paralleled what I had experienced in another dimension. I recall two images of my dying.

During the first, I was in a stream of warm air and floating away from my body. I saw my dead grandmother and told her, "I'm not ready yet." I turned my back against the flow of the warm air, but I still wanted to talk to her. Over my shoulder, I said, "I'm sorry they didn't let me go to your funeral." She replied, "Darling, I've always known. Now go." And then I literally dove back into my body, comforted by an image of friends and family waiting for me.

Some time passed and I sensed I couldn't hold on any longer. I felt like horses were pounding me and I had to let go. At the last minute, I had the sensation of someone pinning me in my body and I thought, "He's holding me. I have to stay."

When I came to, I saw my parents. They'd flown halfway across the country when they heard I'd been brought into emergency and had collapsed. I moved my left hand in circles and my father took that to mean that I wanted a pen. I wrote, "Thanks for coming." As soon as he saw me include the period, my dad said he knew I'd be okay. I never saw his optimism crack.

A week and half later, there was a new emergency. My bile duct was leaking. I had to go back to surgery and be opened up again. A few weeks later, I needed a third surgery as necrotic liver tissue was festering inside me. This time, they went in through the back and my doctor had to remove a rib to be able to properly clean out my thoracic cavity. The space where my rib had been was packed and bandaged.

My doctor was going away for a couple of days, which made me nervous. He assured me I'd be okay and that he'd remove the packing when he came back. He specifically told me not to let anyone take it out until he got back.

Two days later, Halloween to be exact, when my father was downstairs getting a cup of coffee and I was alone in my room, the senior surgical resident came in. He told me he was going to remove the packing from my wound. I remembered my doctor's admonition to keep the packing in and my internal voice that had said "participate!" I explained that Doctor T. had said he didn't want the packing removed and that he'd do it when he returned. The resident's response was, "Well, he's away and I'm in charge." He turned me over, removed the packing, then left my room.

I drifted off. Then I opened my eyes and saw that my entire bed was covered in blood. I was so weak I couldn't reach the call button. When my father came back to my room, he dropped his coffee and ran for the nurses. In the chaos that followed, my feeding tube also got dislodged. I remember general pandemonium . . . people running and others appearing out of nowhere . . . people calling things out to me, to someone. The chaos made me panic. I started to hyperventilate.

The senior surgical resident came back in and was yelling his name at me and telling me to calm down. Seeing him made me panic more. Another resident, Jacques-who-I'll-never-forget, told me to look into his eyes and breathe into a paper bag. He was my friend. He used to come and tell me about his life. I knew him enough to trust him and calm down. The bleeding was staunched, but I had to have several transfusions.

When my doctor returned, he was furious. It turned out he hadn't wanted the packing removed because I was on a blood thinner and he knew that would have to be stopped first. The senior resident came in to apologize, but I couldn't look at him. I was afraid of him from then on.

My father held me together that day. The only thing I had from home was a beautiful blue bathrobe. When I saw that it was also soaked in blood, I felt something inside me dissolve. I said to my father, "Daddy, I don't think I can master this. This is too much for us to handle." His response: "We can handle anything. Don't worry. I guarantee you'll feel better after a couple of hours of sleep." Comforted by his reassurance, I succumbed to my exhaustion. It had been a messy Halloween.

When I woke up, it was barely dawn. I saw my father in the armchair beside my bed and asked him if he'd been there all night. "No," he said, "I went home for a bit." He paused and then said, "I have something for you." And he handed me my bathrobe . . . as clean, clear, and blue as a summer sky, fresh and perfectly ironed. He'd gone home to wash it and was seen ironing it at 5 A.M. There was no residue of any mayhem anywhere I looked. He was drinking his morning coffee. The sun was up. We were fine.

Both of my parents took exquisite, intuitive care of my sense of self, how I viewed my situation, how it all looked from the inside out. My frame of mind was one thing they could actively manage. The bathrobe was important and symbolic to me and so it was to my dad. My physical sense of self was shocked and fragile, and my mother tended to it as she would a newborn.

After the second surgery, two nurses came in to change my dressings and one said to my mother, "It's pretty gruesome. You may want to step outside." I said, "It's okay, Mom. You can come right back after. You don't have to watch." But my mother just looked at me and said, "If you're staying, I'm staying. If I love you, I love your wounds." My long, deep, open wounds never seemed worrisome again, at least not to me.

My parents were a seamless blend of strength and optimism. Their love for me kept me alive as I faced a long tunnel of darkness. Their devotion held me as if transfixed on the path home.

Over ten or twelve weeks, nurses came and went, but there seemed to be too many other lives and deaths around our floor for them to connect to anyone. They told me stories about the guy next door, and then he died. And then more stories about another guy, and then he died. I'm not sure who needed the distance between us more, the nurses or me.

One thing that was memorable was a pending nurses' strike, which made matters worse. One nurse said, "You're a lawyer. I'm sure you understand our concerns. We just have to strike." But her words struck cold fear into me. All I could understand, lawyer or not, was that her serious and dire concerns did not include my welfare in any way. I was hooked up to machines and completely dependent on the hospital staff to live. But I was not on her mind at all. I was petrified. All I could think of was, "If there's a strike, what's going to happen to me?"

I have fond memories of two residents who connected with me as a real person. They'd drop in, ask me how I was doing, and just chat. For example, one of them described his daughter's bumblebee costume that she'd be wearing for Halloween. The other one, Jacques-who-I'll-never-forget, told me about taking someone on a date to see a movie and what the movie had been like. These conversations helped me remember there was a real world out there where people did normal things. These chats linked me to a life I could have beyond the hospital.

Several months after collapsing in emergency, and three operations later, I was scarred, covered in bandages, and incredibly weak, but well enough to go home to recuperate.

My surgeon said, "I want to ask you something unorthodox. There's a whole team of people who have been quietly cheering for you since the first dark days. They want to see you going home, and I want you to meet them." I was dressed to leave the hospital, and so he wheeled me down to the surgical staff lounge.

There were about thirty-five people there, waiting for me. They began clapping and cheering for me. I was dumbfounded. I clapped back to them. I started to cry. Some of them also cried.

My surgeon had been fantastic. He had showed tremendous respect for me as a person. He always made me feel like he spent his whole morning getting ready to see me. Every time I saw him, he'd say, "How's my fighter?" I felt we were partners together in a project and neither of us would let the other down. I certainly would not be letting him down.

I am sure I only survived because of my doctor's great care and my parents' great love. None of them ever let me believe that something couldn't be handled. All three of them were my partners. My parents were also my guardians and my advocates. My doctor was my champion.

"Creepy"

After a month at home, it was time to start rehab. Everyone called me "Creepy" because of how I walked. I couldn't stand up straight and could only shuffle my feet. All the bed rest in the hospital had created a scoliosis in my spine.

I went to rehab every day for five hours, for six months. There were times they would have me do something, like just go up a couple of steps and down again, and I'd have to have a nap. Everything was so tough. Small bags of peanuts were the first weights I lifted.

My mother drove me to rehab every morning at 9:30 and picked me up every afternoon. In the car one day, I remember saying, "I can't go there again. I can't do this again. How am I going to get through this? What am I going to do.?" And she said,

"You just open the door. You just go in. I love you. I have nothing else to say." It must have been so difficult for her to see me working so hard and still struggling so much. She was my rock, and she was steadfast with her love, her support, and her focus. And, of course, I knew what I had to do—"Pamela—participate."

After the six months of rehab, I had regained some strength and some flexibility. But I was not finished. I still had more hurdles to clear.

Maimonides' Prayer

Ten months after my initial emergency collapse, it was determined that I was ready to talk about future reconstructive surgery on my abdomen. It felt really important to me to check out the prospect of minimizing the disfigurement I had suffered. I knew I would need to have some muscles and ribs rearranged, and I also needed some plastic surgery to diminish the magnitude and lumpiness of some very long, very deep, puffy scars, almost like trenches, running at angles deep into my trunk.

I was referred to someone described as the "most famous and very best" plastic surgeon in the country. I can't even begin to describe how excited I was to be traveling 1,500 miles to see this doctor. The fact that I was now well enough to take this trip by myself was huge. And this artist genius was going to put me back into a young woman's body.

At the time, I was thin and pale, and my hair was short. Much of my hair had fallen out in the hospital and was just growing back. Because of my extensive scarring, I couldn't tuck any clothes into my waist, but I dressed up as much as I could. I can still see myself. I wore a big white shirt of my father's and flowery pants with a loose waist.

The Journey of the Green Elephant

The plastic surgeon's office was unlike any I'd ever seen. Tastefully decorated, it had sophisticated furniture, soft classical music, and a wall fountain. I'd never seen one before. I was in a complete state of awe and excited anticipation.

A nurse took me into an interior office. She told me to get undressed, wrap a sheet around myself, and stand up on the footstool in the middle of the room. When the doctor came in, he told me to drop the sheet. He circled around me, asking questions and nodding. Then he stopped, looked at me (the sheet was still on the floor), and said, "I could make you look once again like a beautiful, young woman; I could fix you, but I won't. Your case is covered by medical insurance and the insurance doesn't pay me enough to keep my children in private schools."

A chasm opened up inside of me. I felt I was falling into it. My eyes brimmed with tears. I had to get away from there. As I stood there, completely naked, he said I was not worth his effort.

Subdued and shaken, I got dressed and began to leave his office. As I reached the door, the doctor looked up from his desk, where two ivory tusks on the wall behind him framed him. He asked how I had heard of him. I replied that he had been recommended by my cousin, Dr. X, a physician in the same city. He suddenly became interested and said, "Oh, your cousin is Dr.X? Well, perhaps we should talk." I was incredulous. I knew that I wanted nothing to do with this man.

Many years after this event, my father-in-law quoted a man named Maimonides, who lived in the twelfth century. He was a scholar, philosopher, codifier of laws, and a very thoughtful and famous physician. Maimonides' "Prayer of the Physician" says:

"O Lord . . . Preserve me from the temptation of allowing myself to be influenced in the exercise of my profession by the thirst for gain or the pursuit of glory. Strengthen my heart so that it may be ever ready to serve both poor and rich, both friend and foe, both just and unjust."

My guess is that Maimonides would have been very disappointed by the famous plastic surgeon and my encounter with him.

I Think of That Nurse Every Day

Months later, I was referred to another plastic surgeon. He was extremely competent and very kind. Based on my previous experience, I'd say I actually ended up with the best after all. He even gave me a belly button again.

After the corrective surgery, my doctor left detailed instructions for the nursing staff. He also told me how the bandages that encased my entire torso should be wrapped when the dressings were changed. He was very specific and insistent about the importance of the bandage not only covering my scars, but also that they come down a few inches below the scar line.

My first nurse followed the doctor's instructions and did it perfectly. Hours passed and there was a shift change.

Eventually, I realized my dressings were overdue to be changed. I buzzed for the nurse and asked if they could be done. The new nurse had a chip on her shoulder. Assuming I was in the hospital for a tummy tuck, she said, "I know you're a cosmetic patient—I'll get to you when I get to you."

When this nurse finally did come in, she was cold and nasty and she bound me incorrectly, not taking the bandage down far enough. I asked her if she could please fully cover the scar. I explained that my doctor had been very explicit about how it should be done. She challenged me, saying, "Are you telling me how to do my job? I don't have time to do this again. There are people here with real injuries. My priority is not your tummy tuck."

I was shocked! I was rendered mute by both her callousness and by the worrisome realization that she had worked on me without really reading the chart.

Because of that nurse, I have an ugly bump on my belly, beneath the scars crisscrossing my body. The scars remind me of excellent care and a life saved. The red bump reminds me of someone's bad mood and disdain. I think of that nurse every day. I wish I'd been more forceful with her.

I believe that when you are dealing with an unpleasant sales-clerk at a department store, you're actually in training for the occasional health care professional who seems to be missing the empathy gene. Fortunately, they are in the minority, and I do have faith in the system as a whole.

From Being Healed to Being Saved

While recuperating at home, I saw my family doctor regularly. He would check my progress and sometimes we'd just talk. On one visit, I told him, "I think there's something wrong with my face. It feels a bit paralyzed." He replied that it could be some residual nerve damage, given everything I'd been through, but asked me to tell him again how it felt. I said, "It feels like I have a mask on my face."

He said, "I think you're in a depression. And if anyone has reason for a depression, it would be you. I recommend that you see Dr. Y, a psychiatrist. I think the two of you will have a lot to talk about."

When Life Is Threatened: The Importance of Support

My sessions with Dr. Y were completely liberating. I went through every step of my ordeal with him. I came to understand that I was suffering from post-traumatic stress, something unheard of twenty years ago. I had badly needed to talk about what had happened to me but hadn't wanted to share the details of the awfulness with the people I loved. I had created a protective mask.

This skillful psychiatrist guided me through the last steps of my journey, past being physically healed to being psychologically saved.

After five hours, our conversation comes to a natural close. The green elephant sits there, quietly, as though watching her, bearing witness, having taken everything in.

This woman fully recovered and returned to work. She is now married, has four children and a warm and nourishing home, and has started a school based on "awe and wonder." She is also a talented artist, and the images in her paintings are bold and strong. Her memories of her previous health care experiences, albeit still vivid, are just memories, not daily challenges. Daily challenges now include helping with homework, renovating a house, and finding time as a hospital board member to read a report on "Enhancing the Quality of Patient Care."

I NEEDED A GUIDE

IT WAS A WARM AUGUST NIGHT. It should have been perfect for the fireworks display scheduled to celebrate the city's birthday. But heavy fog had moved in from the harbor, settling in, obscuring the view. The crowds of people began to disperse.

Beth, a single mother, began to walk to the car with her two sons and a couple of children from her neighborhood. Beth's husband, the boys' father, was not there. Richard, an emergency room physician and orthopedic surgeon, had died a year earlier as a result of liver cancer.

There were hundreds of people about, all moving toward cars and home. Several were crossing a wide boulevard using the pedestrian crosswalk.

Then there was a terrible sound—a thud—the sound of a car connecting with a human body. Beth's younger son, Adam, had been hit by a car traveling too fast. The driver was oblivious to the crowds of people and to the crosswalk sign. The driver was oblivious because the driver was drunk.

The ambulance arrived before Beth knew it, and her son was sped off to the hospital, with Beth following behind in a police car. Paul, Adam's brother and Beth's older son, was to go to a friend's house and wait for her there.

At the hospital, a social worker greeted Beth as she walked through the door. In Beth's words, "This was the most important element of the care I received at the hospital." She continues:

Hospitals are very strange places under the best of circumstances. In a serious emergency situation, you need a guide. You're in shock and need hand-holding, someone to help your mind work, to see what you can do, and then help you do it. You basically need to borrow a working mind. You have to make decisions. Someone has to help you see what decisions are to be made. This social worker filled this need for me. She had lost family, too, and she understood. Not only was she a godsend that night, she also stayed in touch with me for several weeks, which was a comfort.

The second most important need Beth had was for information. She desperately wanted to know what was going on. She did know that Adam had been taken immediately to the operating room, but that was all she knew. As it turned out, a friend, an orthopedic surgeon who just happened to be in the hospital that night, facilitated communication between the operating room and the small, private room where Beth was waiting.

This friend was able to give Beth an indication that things were not going well. It helped, she said, to have some warning of the cruel reality that was to follow. "My mind had been fighting against the worst possibilities. I'd been thinking we could go home soon. I realized I needed to shift my thinking and to get ready for the truth—that we wouldn't be going home, that Adam would never be coming home."

Beth had a very strong network of family and friends. Because there was a phone in the room where she was waiting, she was able to call people, to put them on alert, to ask them for help, to find out where her other son was, and to begin to make arrangements when the final, tragic truth of Adam's death was finally relayed to her.

I Needed A Guide

The physician who had been in the operating room, desperately trying to save Adam's life, offered to speak to Beth's son Paul at any time. He knew that Paul might want or need to try to piece together what happened after his brother had been rushed away in the ambulance.

The guidance of the social worker and her follow-up calls, the communication flow to ease the burden of waiting in ignorance or in fantasy, the support of friends, and the offers for follow-up conversations kept Beth going. She says, "I do not know how awful this horrific situation would be for someone who is not in her home town or for someone who speaks another language or for someone who is socially isolated."

Beth had to endure reliving this trauma through the court case that ensued. The driver of the car that hit and killed Adam was found to be guilty of driving under the influence of alcohol. Beth and Paul have both spoken publicly about the powerful effects of combining alcohol and driving.

RISE & SHINE

In early April, my wife, Bertha, had a biopsy of a breast lump that had come and gone for several months. Its erratic nature, combined with delays in the medical system, meant that Bertha kept missing the window for testing. After the biopsy was done, we were told that if there was a problem, we'd hear in two or three days. It was really hard to focus. We were both like robots at work, there in body but not in mind. At home, we'd often just wander around the house. We tried to distract ourselves with novels but couldn't concentrate.

We were on pins and needles for the first seventy-two hours, but, as the days passed without a phone call, we both began to relax. We presumed everything was okay. We noticed that the sun was shining again.

On April 20, Bertha went to our regular family doctor for a routine appointment. Because there was no reason to do otherwise, I didn't go with her. She went alone.

When Bertha walked into the doctor's office, just at the beginning of the appointment, her doctor handed her a brochure titled, "How to Deal with Breast Cancer." Bertha read between the lines immediately. Obviously, a phone call that should have been made in the initial seventy-two hours after the biopsy had somehow been overlooked. Our family doctor, thinking he was being helpful, with a simple gesture, had pulled the ground out from under our feet.

The implied news that the lump had been malignant was completely unanticipated. Of course, Bertha was devastated. And when I finally found out what had happened, I was overcome not just with fear, but also with an enormous sense of guilt that Bertha had had to hear this news alone. I should have been with her!

Rise & Shine

As Bertha tried to absorb the fact that she had breast cancer and had to have surgery, I felt completely helpless. I felt the very center of our lives being threatened. There was only the tiniest sense of comfort that Bertha was going to get the medical help she needed. Quite legitimately, Bertha was being treated as the patient, but I felt I was also caught in the whirlwind of this terrifying illness. I needed to know what I could do. I needed a meaningful role to play. None was suggested by any doctor.

After Bertha's surgery, while waiting for her chemotherapy to begin, an idea began to form in my mind. I thought Bertha needed a smile, even if just for a second, and so I began to search through books for special sayings or quotations that might boost her spirits. It became a way for me to help her, to give her some encouragement, to say "you can do this!"

Bertha's chemotherapy started on June 10 and so did my found quotes—the first one was "Damn the torpedoes, full steam ahead!" (Admiral David Farragut). I always left the quotes on the kitchen table. I specifically left them there because it meant that Bertha had a reason to get out of bed each morning to see them. It gave her something to start her day.

I know they mattered to her. She said, in a recent speech she gave, "The quotes were a bright spot in my day. I'd stick them up all around the house—in the kitchen, in the bathroom, beside my pillow—wherever I might need some encouragement. I put some up beside my copy of 'Warnings of Possible Reactions to Chemotherapy.' The quotes served as a countermeasure to the dreadful reality I was dealing with. Some of them are still up on my mirror even now. One can always use some motivation!"

These daily gifts to my beloved wife also helped me deal with my own private pain and agonizing sense of helplessness.

Through it all, I got the satisfaction that I was doing something. I was helping Bertha cope. In a way, it was no big deal, but it worked for both of us.

It doesn't make me any kind of hero. In fact, this whole cancer journey has changed my thoughts about heroes. I used to think that people like Winston Churchill were my heroes, but I've changed my view. It's the people on the cancer wards—the nurses, doctors, and pharmacists, and the women who are fighting breast cancer—they're my heroes now!

———————

Bertha and her husband, Wayne, gave this collection of quotes to the Canadian Breast Cancer Foundation to use as a fundraiser and to boost the spirits of others who journey in crisis. The collection was published under the title of Rise & Shine. *A second volume of 180 quotes will be released this year (2006). Bertha continues in remission, and Wayne hopes that a cure for breast cancer will be found.*

A PROFOUNDLY
ISOLATING EXPERIENCE

MAGGIE HOLDS HER COFFEE CUP. She is simply and neatly dressed and she looks completely composed. She starts talking, in a calm, soft-spoken manner. It is clear she has given this interview a lot of thought. Her words come slowly, somewhat haltingly. And then she stops and apologizes for what she describes as "being so dumb." She adds, "I think I've processed all of this, but my hands are shaking."

She closes her eyes and rubs her temples and forehead, as if to carefully retrieve the ten-year journey of her husband's illness. It's been seven years since Richard died.

Before she goes any further, Maggie stresses that she does not want to name or blame. "I'm grateful to all the people who cared for Richard. They did the best they could. I know that all health care professionals mean well." She is so gracious and repeats this sentiment many times during the next two hours.

Richard's nosebleeds began in 1988, two and a half years after Maggie and Richard were married. At that time, they had a one-year-old, and Maggie was pregnant with their second child. They were living in a suburb of a large city, far away from both of their families.

Richard traveled a lot and thought that possibly his nosebleeds were being caused by the dry air of long airplane flights. One of his nosebleeds occurred while he was in Germany and was so bad he had to be hospitalized. The bleeding stopped and he was able to fly home, but he realized it was time to go see a doctor.

Richard ended up being referred to an ear, nose, and throat specialist. He didn't see any need for Maggie to come to his appointments with him. Initially, she didn't give this a second thought, in part because it would have been difficult with a one-year-old and no babysitters.

The specialist decided that Richard should have exploratory surgery to try to determine what was causing the nosebleeds. "Maybe Richard knew that the surgery was, in fact, a biopsy, but that word was never mentioned to me. Nonetheless, I wanted to be at the hospital when the doctor spoke to my husband about what he found out during surgery. I couldn't contact the doctor at the hospital and so I kept calling his office to say—'I'm home with a young baby and can't wait at the hospital all day. Please just ask the doctor to let me know when he's going to talk to Richard and I can get there in thirty minutes.'"

Either the doctor never got the message or he didn't think it was important for Maggie to be there when he told Richard that surgery had revealed a cancerous mass that looked like adenoid cystic carcinoma.

Maggie did accompany Richard to a follow-up appointment with this doctor to learn about what was in store for her husband. The doctor walked into the office and said, "Hi Richard, would your wife mind leaving the room?"

Maggie recalls, "I can't believe it, but I did leave the room. I felt so angry and so vulnerable and so intimidated. I think the doctor just wanted a very clinical experience and was afraid I'd demonstrate some sort of emotion. But he didn't even know me. In fact, I hardly ever cry and never in public. He was shutting me out of my own life for reasons that weren't valid in my case.

A Profoundly Isolating Experience

"Richard, too, kept a certain distance after the initial stage of treatment, saying he didn't need me to go to his appointments with him. I think he needed to feel some control when things were so out of control. Whenever I asked about the appointments, he didn't tell me very much. I was young, pregnant, and far away from family and friends. I couldn't get my questions answered directly by anyone."

Two weeks after the diagnosis, Richard was scheduled for surgery to remove the tumor. The operation was supposed to take place at 8 A.M., but the surgeon did not arrive until 2 P.M. By that time, Richard was not only hungry and impatient, but he'd also had a long time to think about his work and upcoming commitments. Apparently, he asked his surgeon if he would be able to attend a meeting in Toronto the following week.

Maggie learned about this because the same doctor who had asked her to leave his office ten days earlier now called her at home immediately after Richard's surgery. Maggie describes that he sounded furious as he said, "Your husband just asked me if he can travel next week. Clearly, you guys aren't taking this seriously. This isn't the flu. This will likely travel to his brain and kill him."

"That was all he said. I just looked at the phone after he hung up. There had been no kindness in his voice, only irritation. I had seen my grandfather die slowly, stroke after stroke, and I suddenly saw what was likely ahead of me. I kept this horrifying reality to myself. I never told anyone about the doctor's call."

For the next three years, Richard had lots of radiation and continued to work and go to his doctor's appointments alone. Any information Maggie had was through Richard, secondhand. Life just went on.

But Maggie started to notice that one of Richard's eyes didn't look right. She'd tell Richard, "I think there's something different about your eye. Please tell your doctor that your wife is concerned and that she thinks you should have a CT scan. And Richard would come back from an appointment and say, 'The doctor thinks I only need one CT scan a year and I'm not scheduled for one for several months.'"

"No one was listening to my concerns, including Richard's ophthalmologist. But eventually, his eye looked so strange that anyone could tell from looking at him that something was terribly wrong." What happened next was a turning point for Maggie.

After nine months, Richard finally had his regularly scheduled CT scan. Maggie continues her story:

The doctor called both of us in and told Richard, "You have a problem I can't deal with, and I'm going to refer you to a head and neck specialist." And he gave us Richard's file to take to the new doctor. I read it from cover to cover, including the report from the radiologist that spelled out, in words even I could understand, that there was a huge and new tumor. Clearly, there'd been an unnecessary lag in diagnosis. You'd think an eye doctor would have been concerned that Richard's eye had been showing lots of vascular activity for months. And after three years of following Richard, this doctor didn't have the guts to tell us what had been found. He just passed us off.

You want to believe that doctors will fix everything. But sometimes they're not paying attention or don't know or admit to the limitations of their own expertise. I learned the hard way. It took this brutal experience to make me assert myself and get involved. I told Richard that I'd be coming to his appointments and that I'd be speaking up and that he needed to get ready.

We went to see the new head and neck doctor together. He was a kind, older man who told Richard, in complicated medical language, that the cancer had spread to his eye and would require surgery. Because I had lived with my sister, who is an orthoptist, I understood some "medicalese." I also knew from reading the file that Richard had had a recurrence and that when the doctors talked about "treatment," that meant that Richard would lose his eye. But they were using such complex language that Richard had to ask, "Will the surgery affect my eye?"

I concluded that it was this doctor's own humanity that kept him from spelling things out or preparing us for the tough realities we would be facing. It was as though he wanted to protect us and thought that if he just asked us how our Thanksgiving was and didn't tell us things, we wouldn't worry. I also think he was uncomfortable with the situation himself, but if you can't communicate bad news, then why go into medicine?

Richard's eye was removed. And over the following six years, he had nine more operations.

It was like my husband was chained to a radiator and couldn't escape the invisible monster living in the house who fed on Richard's flesh. The monster would come out now and then and take pieces of him, but the experts didn't want to talk to us about the situation. We wanted to know when the monster was likely to come out again, and how they would deal with it, but it was as though the doctors would merely say, "Don't worry! We're the monster tamers. We'll take care of everything."

But not having specific information did not keep me from worrying. If you don't know what to worry about specifically, then you worry about everything. My imagination worked overtime, especially at night. I conjured up horrible things and often felt like I was living out my nighttime fears during the day.

On top of everything else, our new baby had very bad asthma, the kind where they don't ask you for any information when you run into emergency but just grab your child and start treatment. At home, I had to give him medicine every four hours. I had to keep him alive. I didn't get enough sleep. I coped, but I was depressed. I shut down. In hindsight, I missed our baby's infancy.

Richard's surgeries left him horrifically disfigured. It was a profoundly isolating experience. I couldn't appreciate what it was like to be in Richard's shoes, he couldn't appreciate what it was like to be in my shoes, and no one could appreciate what it was like to be in our shoes.

While Richard seemed to handle everything magnificently, we didn't really talk about things. It was only after he died, when I was going through all the papers in his desk, that I found something he'd written that conveyed how isolated he had felt.

Of course, the kids were affected by all this as well. Our baby, when he was two, drew pictures of eyes everywhere and would go around the house chanting, "First Daddy had two eyes, and then he had one." Our three-year-old understood that the doctors had used a knife to take his daddy's eye away and quietly concluded they could take everything away and that his dad could disappear completely.

I can't tell you how many times I felt like I was supposed to just sit in a corner like a golden retriever and smile. It was as though I was wallpaper. A group of physicians would come into a tiny examining room and introduce themselves to Richard and completely ignore me. I wanted to scream, "Didn't you have mothers? Weren't you taught manners?" But I didn't scream, because I wanted the staff to like my husband. It was a difficult balancing act—"be nice, but make sure Richard gets what he needs."

There was a time when Richard was in a horrible state. By then I knew his situation so well I could tell he was facing a crisis and, if something wasn't done, he would die. His doctor had dismissed his problems as a cold. I took him to the emergency room and told the staff that he had to be seen and I wasn't going home. The doctors finally agreed that Richard's condition was not only serious, it was very grave. He needed major brain and facial reconstructive surgery. It took three days to put together a team of ten surgeons to perform the fourteen-hour operation.

I suppose this whole situation could have been intimidating, but I was beyond intimidation. I knew I had to do what I could to keep him alive. Richard wouldn't advocate for himself. I know that I saved his life that day by being so fierce.

When asked if there were any positive memories about Richard's care, Maggie immediately says:

> Above all, I'm grateful for everything that everyone did. They gave us ten years. But there are three doctors who stand out, and two of them were part of the team who helped Richard through that particular crisis.
>
> As each member of the team was found, the doctors, one by one, came in to meet Richard. One of them arrived a bit later than he'd said, and the first words out of his mouth were, "Sorry to keep you waiting." In ten years, he was the only one who ever said that! And when I asked him if he'd ever done this operation before, he didn't flinch from the question but spoke the truth. He said, "I've done a dozen other operations with this level of complexity, but I've never done exactly this. We'll be making this up as we go." I appreciated his honesty.
>
> Another of the doctors came in and introduced himself to both of us (rare in itself). Then he asked Richard how old he was (thirty-seven), where he lived (a nearby suburb), and whether he had any children (two). Through these three simple questions, this doctor communicated that he understood there was a whole human being in the bed. I almost wept, because this doctor was acknowledging his shared humanity with my husband. This was incredibly important to me at that time, and I'll never forget this man.

A Profoundly Isolating Experience

The third doctor who was special was the one Richard had during his last year. The doctor who had followed Richard for six years called us into his office and said, with tears in his eyes, "Go home and live your life." This was his way of saying, "There's nothing more to be done." But we pressed for another answer and ended up with a wonderful oncologist who bravely took on Richard's case. He always asked Richard, "What have you noticed?" Then he would ask me, too. He spoke clearly and honestly and with genuine kindness. He sought out treatment options and coordinated Richard's care. I no longer felt that I was Richard's sole case manager. It felt like the three of us were together in this very difficult situation. And when Richard was dying, this doctor came and made his own private goodbye. He quietly and soundlessly just held Richard's foot. It meant a lot to me that he was invested enough to do that.

The palliative care team was incredibly helpful at the most difficult time. It amazes me that people choose to put themselves daily in the way of such suffering, and I will always be grateful for their deep compassion and understanding.

Six months after Richard's death, I wrote the hospital to advocate for some kind of extra support for other people dealing with similar circumstances. It's not just the disease that needs to be treated; the whole person and the whole family need help knowing how they are to live in the world. There wasn't even a support group at the hospital. I believe that psychological support should be standard care for patients having drastic facial surgery, and that the hospital has a responsibility to make sure patients get it. A gifted psychiatrist can form a connection with someone very quickly to help reduce the sense of isolation. Even a chance to talk openly while the patient is still postoperative would make a big difference. But the hospital was very resistant to these ideas. This was so sad, because there's so much for hospitals to learn from asking patients and families about their experiences.

Maggie noted, weeks after telling her story for this book, that "One of my children just had an appointment at the local children's hospital, and I saw a notice by the reception desk that said patient advocates were available if you needed help. In all the ten years of Richard being followed by his hospital, I never heard of such a person as a patient advocate or of anyone else who could facilitate solutions to some of the problems we were having with health care delivery."

HIS NAME MEANS
"RISE ABOVE THE STORM"

IT WAS A DARK AND STORMY NIGHT.

The weather system that started that February day in 2004 would eventually be called a weather bomb, and record books would be rewritten. In a twenty-four-hour period, this blizzard's devastating combination of 95.5 centimeters (37.6 inches) of snow and gale-force winds of 124 kilometers (77.5 miles) per hour created snowdrifts so deep and so high you could ski down them.

The province of Nova Scotia declared a state of emergency. It was as though everyone and everything was encased in a white cocoon. For most people, nothing moved for days. For a young couple and their young son, however, an extraordinary drama began to unfold at the height of the storm, after the power went out.

Kim was actually excited when she heard a storm was coming. She figured the snow would prevent her husband, Scott, from working his usual twelve-hour day as a contractor. While they needed him to work to pay their debts, she thought it would be fun to have him home for the day and that he would enjoy playing with their son, Milo, who was almost two and loved snow. It was going to be a good day. She was cooking a nice ham dinner, and her favorite TV show, *ER*, was on that night. Kim smiled to herself.

Scott and Milo did have fun outside. Among other things, even though the truck was low on gas, they drove it back and forth, trying to beat down tracks to keep their driveway open. Scott figured he'd be getting lots of calls for additional work as soon as the snow stopped. Eventually, though, there was so much snow, the truck got stuck.

Around 6 P.M., Kim started to feel a bit "off." She was six months pregnant and thought the baby was giving her indigestion. She and Scott had dinner and put Milo to bed. Outside, the storm intensified; inside, Kim's discomfort and Scott's concern also intensified. By midnight, when the power went out and they lost phone service, they knew they were in trouble. Kim was scared; Scott figured he had to get her to the hospital.

Scott started shoveling like a madman. All he had was a child's shovel, and it wasn't long enough to get under the truck. Scott, remarkably clever for his twenty-four years, rigged up a bar across the door to their house and winched the truck backward. Meanwhile, Kim was inside, lighting candles and trying to stay calm between contractions.

After three hours, Scott managed to get their truck to the top of their driveway. Only then did he and Kim wake up their son, dress him for the trip into the city, and put him in the truck. Disturbed from a deep sleep, Milo was disoriented and frightened. Kim's cries of pain, when she had contractions, frightened him even more.

Scott and Kim lived outside the city, near the famous Peggy's Cove Lighthouse. Under normal circumstances, the drive from their house to the city took about thirty-five minutes and was one of the most beautiful in the world, curving back and forth alongside the ocean's edge, past picturesque fishing harbors. The drive this night, though, would be completely different. All highways were officially closed. There was no visibility, and the snow was so deep that Scott knew he would have to drive fast to maintain enough momentum to get through the drifts. He knew he had to keep the truck moving, because if the truck stopped, he would not be able to get it going again. But it wasn't driving fast on a twisting road during a raging blizzard that frightened Scott. It was the truck's gas light indicator being on that terrified him.

Miraculously, not only was Scott able to handle the truck on the unplowed roads and make it scale enormous drifts, he also found a gas station open that, while it had no staff present, still had power, meaning that its pumps were still working. Even more astounding to Scott, given the state of their finances, was that his credit card was accepted.

All during the terrifying and dangerous drive, Kim was in a state of disbelief that she could be in labor. She thought, "I'm only twenty-four weeks. It's too early." Scott, on the other hand, had concluded and fully accepted that Kim was having a miscarriage, but he kept this thought to himself. He just focused on what he viewed as his job and only responsibility, which was getting Kim to the hospital. He didn't know it yet, but he'd find out that much more was in store for them both.

Kim, Scott, and Milo arrived at the hospital between 4 and 5 A.M. Kim was examined and rushed into a birthing room. Her contractions were close. Scott wanted to stay with her but first wanted to settle Milo back to sleep in his portable crib in the next room, because Kim's cries kept waking him up. But the hospital staff said Milo could only stay if he stayed in the same room with them.

Scott was incredulous. "The hospital was not busy, and I knew Milo would just go to sleep if he was given half a chance. There are times when policies should be lapsed. It was a miracle we had all arrived in one piece, and now I was being told I had to go back out in that storm and risk my life and Milo's all over again." But Scott felt he had no choice but to gather Milo up and head back to his truck.

As luck would have it, Scott's younger brother had an apartment in the city six or seven blocks away, so Scott headed in that direction. He got as close as he could and had to leave the truck in the middle of a road. His brother's street, narrow and steep, was impassable. Scott and Milo were going to have to walk up the hill. The problem was that the snow was up to Scott's waist. He knew there was no way Milo could walk, yet Scott couldn't carry him and move himself, too. Scott grabbed a blanket from the truck, tied Milo in, and pulled the blanket behind him. Scott remembers: "My poor brother—he was woken at five in the morning as I handed him a screaming baby. My brother had been asleep for hours and had no idea what was going on outside."

Meanwhile, back at the hospital, while Scott was dealing with Milo, Kim was trying to communicate with a nurse. She recalls, "This nurse kept talking to me, rambling on with horrible statistics, telling me my baby was going to be born dead and that they were not going to resuscitate it. I started crying. I kept saying, 'I need a doctor. I need my husband.' The nurse countered with, 'A doctor isn't going to change anything. I'm telling you the truth.' I decided I just wasn't going to have this baby even though I was seven centimeters dilated. I remember wondering if she wasn't taking me seriously, because I looked really young and had arrived wearing big boots, pajama bottoms, and a long shirt."

When Scott got back to the hospital, he realized that Kim was distraught and completely overwhelmed.

> I got hold of a doctor who spelled out the situation.
> He explained there was a 60 percent chance the baby

would be stillborn, and I would have to decide whether the baby should be resuscitated. Then the doctor told me that even if the baby was successfully revived, there would be a significant risk of cerebral palsy and/or blindness. I knew I didn't want that for our child.

The hardest thing for me was to be faced with these kinds of choices. Kim was beyond being able to make decisions. I knew I would have to do this alone. I felt I couldn't make the decision, and so I decided to let our baby decide. If he wanted to live, he would.

At 7:17 A.M., our son was born, and he let out a squawk right away. I was so relieved, because the decision had been taken out of my hands. Because he was born at twenty-four weeks and five days and only weighed one pound, twelve ounces, we were told that there was only a slim chance that he would survive more than a couple of hours or days. I thought, "Well, he's come this far. Let's see what he decides to do."

Kim picked up the story. "When he was born, they laid him on my belly for the briefest second, and then we didn't see him again for several hours. The sight of him was scary. He looked like an alien. It was so hard to see a part of us in that state."

Scott jumped back in, saying, "We named him right away. We wanted to make sure that, if he lived, everyone would know who to root for. We picked the name Eli Storm, because Eli means 'rise above' and, taken together, Eli Storm seemed to be strong. We thought he both deserved and needed a fighting name.

"Eli had to have heart surgery at two weeks of age. It was a frightening time for us. One thing that helped was a bulletin board they have on the unit with pictures of other babies who'd been there, and pictures of them now with little stories about them. These faces gave me hope that Eli could have a future."

Scott thought back to the four months that Eli was in the hospital and admitted that he was largely detached. "Because I had concluded, as we drove in to the hospital on the night of the storm, that Kim was having a miscarriage, it was hard for me to let myself fall in love with this little guy when he was born. Also, Eli didn't want to be held or cuddled, and so I pretty much stayed detached and went back to work. We already had huge debts and now had new expenses like gas and a car for Kim to get back and forth to the hospital. We were in desperate financial shape, and I had to work all the time. I couldn't visit except maybe one day a week. Working so hard, in part, was how I coped."

While Scott worked almost nonstop, Kim was going back and forth to visit Eli in the hospital. She explained:

> I knew I wanted to breast-feed Eli when he came home, whenever that would be, and so I pumped the whole time he was in the hospital. For the last month of the four months he was there, I was able to actually nurse him two to three times a day.
>
> I visited Eli every day. I almost always had to go alone. Scott was working all the time, and anyone else who might have been able to come with me had to stay at home and look after Milo. Milo wasn't particularly welcome in the NICU because he wanted to touch everything.
>
> But even though I went to the hospital every day, I wouldn't really do anything when I got there. Most days, I would just sit there. Often I would leave the blanket over

His Name Means "Rise Above the Storm"

Eli's incubator because it bothered me to look at him. He looked so weird. The few times family members came in to see him, I was almost embarrassed about how he looked.

The nurses were wonderful. A number of them really bonded with Eli, and I was so grateful to them. Eli's nurses always made daily and nightly entries about him in a hand-written journal they gave to me when we left the hospital. On Mother's Day, they gave me a series of framed Polaroid pictures they'd taken of him at different times. That was so sweet.

One nurse always came to me and touched my shoulder or my hand and asked me, "How are you doing today?" But I'm a very private person and I didn't really let anyone in. Some of the other mothers in the unit tried to get me to talk. I'd listen to them and I liked knowing that many of them were feeling the same way I was. But I didn't want to talk. I felt that if I talked or cried, everything I was trying to keep at arm's length would become real.

Kim and Scott recalled that they were excited to get Eli home, but things were still not easy, and they both admitted to continued feelings of detachment. Kim filled in some of the details:

Eli was on oxygen at home, which made him unhappy and interfered with his sleep. Scott was working nonstop and couldn't help much with the boys. Milo was potty-training and needed my attention, but Eli's care took so much time that I had little left over. Milo wanted to play outside, but I couldn't take Eli out. And I was unhappy, so my family and friends didn't particularly want to be around me. I felt very isolated.

When Life Is Threatened: The Importance of Support

I was depressed and kept trying to say to friends and family, and to both my doctor and Eli's doctor, that I was unhappy. But everyone had an excuse for how I was feeling. They'd say things like, "It's normal to feel a little down with all that you've been through," or they'd try to reassure me by saying, "You're going to be fine—just give it some time." I felt dismissed. No one took me seriously when I said I needed help. I started to think that how I was feeling was all in my head.

In hindsight, I realize I needed help even when Eli was still in the hospital. It would have been good to have had someone raise and address emotional issues with us. We were told where the social worker's office was located, and that we could go talk to her, but we are private people and are not likely, on our own initiative, to go talk to a stranger. I wish she had approached us.

Kim and Scott both agreed that Eli's happiness and their happiness and attachment to him happened over time and in steps. Scott said, "Eli began to sleep better as soon as he came off oxygen. His sleeping well meant that we could sleep well. The next leap forward came when Eli started crawling. He was so delighted to be able move around and discover things. We have started to see him as a jovial person. He still doesn't love to cuddle or be held, but it's so much easier to relax and enjoy him, as he has become more relaxed and able to enjoy life himself." And Kim added, "I just had him at the doctor's for a checkup. He's doing really well on all the things they measure. He's big and healthy and happy. He has completely settled into our family and has become a best friend to his older brother."

~

Natural Allies:
Partnerships in Care

"Most of us feel better when we are seen
and met with authentic presence and regard,
without condescension or contrived intimacy.
We feel good when we are treated as capable,
when we are related to as if we have the capacity
to actually undertake the hardest work in the world,
when a lot is being asked of us, but in ways
that build on our own intrinsic capacities and intelligences."
—*Jon Kabat-Zinn*

"I need to be a collaborator in my care."
—*Kathleen Hipwell*

"The man who goes alone can start today;
but he who travels with another
must wait until the other is ready."
—*Thoreau*

~

It has been said that true involvement of patients and families leads to better, safer, more compassionate clinical care and better clinical outcomes. Why then would anyone not want to deliver or receive care that is as collaborative as it can be?

In the complex world of health care, why would anyone want or think they could do any of it alone? Is not the provision of individualized information, support, and cooperation a two-way street? Are decisions about treatments and procedures made in partnership not better than those determined in isolation?

And, when patients and families offer their observations in a spirit of wanting to make things better for others, why would this ever be refused?

WE ARE NOT VISITORS IN HER LIFE
SOMETHING'S WRONG—PLEASE LISTEN TO ME
THAT'S WHAT WE'RE HERE FOR
WHEN THE BRAIN IS BROKEN
IT TAKES A TEAM
INVESTING IN INFORMATION
IT JUST COMES NATURALLY
AWASH IN DISAPPOINTMENT

WE ARE NOT VISITORS IN HER LIFE

MY MOTHER WAS IN THE EMERGENCY DEPARTMENT OF A COMMUNITY HOSPITAL. She had broken her hip a month earlier and had been discharged. However, she was still somewhat disoriented, and we were concerned about possible cardiac complications. We wanted her admitted to the step-down unit.

My wife and I stayed with her for more than eight hours in emergency. A stream of staff, mostly kind and competent, provided care. My mother was unable to answer some of their questions, and so we supplied needed information and served as her advocates.

It was very fortunate that we were there for her encounter with the cardiologist. He came in and asked, "Who is your cardiologist?" We explained that my mother didn't have a cardiologist. He replied, with a tone of sarcasm, "Well, who put in her pacemaker in 1987 then?" We informed him that she didn't have a pacemaker and that perhaps he had the wrong patient. With no apology or explanation, he left to find the right patient. My mother would never have been able to sort through the confusion between the doctor's assumptions and her reality.

Eventually, my mother was transferred to the step-down unit. Two nurses—new faces—escorted us to the unit where another nurse greeted us. When we asked to stay with my mother as she was being settled in her room, we were told that we could not and were directed to the visitors' room down the hall. I replied, saying, "But we are not visitors in her life!"

My wife explained that she was a nurse, that my mother was easily confused in unfamiliar settings, and that we could help them settle her. She assured the nurses we would not get in their way. Other nurses came out of their patients' rooms, circling us as "the difficult family." Their reply was a firm "no!"

The door to my mother's room was shut and the blinds were lowered. When we were finally allowed to enter her room, we were told that we must be brief, because visiting hours were over for the night. The nurse handed us a pamphlet stating that visiting hours would begin at 11 A.M. the next day.

We had prevented a potential error in the emergency room when a physician began to examine the wrong patient. Why couldn't these nurses see that we were important to my mother's sense of comfort and that we could help them assure the quality and safety of her care?

SOMETHING'S WRONG—
PLEASE LISTEN TO ME!

I'M ONLY TWENTY-FOUR, BUT I FIGURE I'M NEVER GOING TO HAVE A HORRIBLE ILLNESS BECAUSE I'VE DONE MY SUFFERING. Life cannot ever be as bad as it was two years ago.

As I look back, I'd say my problems began when I started junior high school. Up to that time, I had lived in a protected bubble at home. For example, for grades five and six, my parents paid me $300 a year if I didn't watch any TV. When I got to junior high, I realized there was a whole world I didn't know about, and I rebelled.

My rebellion manifested in a variety of forms. In grade seven, I became depressed and bulimic, and I started cutting myself. I'm really smart, but I only passed my year with Cs and Ds. My parents chose to take no action.

In grade eight, I got more depressed. I refused to go to school, complaining that I had headaches. I had a CT scan and was told there was nothing wrong with me. I failed my academic year but was put through anyway. Grade nine was the same story—I dropped out and failed.

In the fall of my grade ten year, a social worker came to our house. I wasn't going to school at all and, officially, I was considered "a truant." I remember sitting on the couch, talking to the social worker and starting to cry uncontrollably.

I was admitted to the child psychiatry unit. Clearly, I was depressed and pretty sick. But, even though I was there for six weeks, no one caught on to the bulimia. They only noticed the cutting because I actually cut a vein. Before I was discharged, I signed a contract with my parents in which I agreed to take

Prozac for three dollars a day. I was also supposed to go to a school for truant kids.

That school terrified me. The other kids were bad, violent, and into sex and drugs. I'd never even kissed anyone. I refused to do any work and stopped taking the Prozac. I became manic, and when I'm manic, I get violent. I was sent back to the psychiatric unit.

I was basically in and out of the hospital for the next two years. When I was seventeen and about to be discharged, it was determined that it wasn't safe for me to go home because I had threatened my parents. Instead, I was sent to a supervised home for adolescents. I hated it and refused to unpack. I only stayed for a day and a half and cried all the time. I was convinced that I didn't belong there and stomped back to the hospital with my bags.

I had exhausted my options. I still couldn't go home, and so, at age seventeen, I became the youngest person ever accepted into the apartment program of Metro Community Housing, which provides appropriate supports for people with intellectual/physical challenges to help them live independently. In my case, I was provided with an apartment, a case worker, and a social worker. I was also given financial support for living costs.

I was really excited about the idea of having my own apartment. But then I moved in. I quickly realized that I was a spoiled brat. I'd always had everything done for me, and I didn't know how to look after myself. I didn't know how to clean, how to manage money, or how to cook—I couldn't even fry an egg. I had an apartment, but—overnight—I was poor and I was completely alone. It was all quite a shock.

Eventually, I moved in with my best friend, who was also receiving disability assistance. We soon realized that what seemed like a great idea wasn't going to work, and our relationship began to unravel. I learned to love vacuuming because I could throw temper tantrums and say terrible things about her without her hearing. It wasn't the best situation, but we coped at a certain level for awhile. And we drank a lot . . . a lot.

Time passed. There were good times and bad times. And then there were terrible, terrible times. Without question, 2003 was the worst year of my life.

For years, I'd been diagnosed as having "bipolar disorder NOS." This is a brain-chemical disorder and can be well managed with medication. At the start of 2003, I was on a medication that was enabling me to do well; I was starting to visit Laing House, a drop-in program for young people living with mental illness.

In January 2003, my psychiatrist made a decision that seemed to be out of the blue and without any logical basis, but with huge consequences. Even though this doctor had been treating me for two years and knew I was making progress, she decided that my diagnosis didn't fit and that most of my issues were caused because I was mostly "borderline."

At first, this notion of being "borderline" appealed to me, because it meant that maybe I could get well by just changing the things I had difficulty with through therapy. Maybe I wouldn't need medication. Also, I presumed my doctor knew what she was doing. I quickly realized, though, that what she was really telling me with this new diagnosis was that I was completely responsible for my symptoms and that I was manipulative, dishonest, and overly dramatic to get attention.

My doctor decided to reduce my medication. I've been prescribed lots of medications over the years, and I've learned the hard way that it's not easy or simple to find a combination that works. Some medications have made me hallucinate or have given me slurred speech or twitches, or have affected my weight. I want to be well, but not with uncomfortable or unhealthy side effects. As my sense of myself started to change, I told my doctor that I was starting to feel really hyper and was having trouble sleeping. She didn't seem concerned.

I'm prone to becoming hypomanic, and I could feel this starting to happen. The sensations of being manic are fun, but I also fear them. I know that when I'm manic, I get violent and don't make appropriate decisions.

In June, while playing softball with my friends at the drop-in center, I was hit in the head by the ball. I had four fractures in the bones around my eye socket and developed a retinal hematoma. I didn't feel any pain because damage to a nerve left most of the left half of my face completely numb. Because I was also hypomanic by this time, I was amused by the whole thing. Standing there, feeling wonderful, and looking at my CT scan—which showed the bones that didn't meet and the giant protruding black blob of air that I'd blown into my eye socket by blowing my nose—was just so surreal. The ophthalmologist said I was the happiest patient he'd ever seen. The next sequence of events, inconsequential in isolation but deadly in combination, created a crisis.

I was supposed to have an early appointment with the eye doctor. I wasn't sleeping much anyway, but that night I made sure I didn't sleep because I was afraid of missing the early appointment. Because I didn't sleep, I didn't take the medications I usually take before I go to bed. To make matters worse, because of the injury, I had had to take some antibiotics for two weeks that had given me severe diarrhea and vomiting for thirteen days.

This meant that any medication I was taking wasn't being kept down.

I'd been sick for thirteen days and knew I was in trouble. I tried to get admitted to the hospital because I could feel myself becoming out of control. I was told that I was okay.

Of course, I think I'm a genius when I'm manic. I'd been reading about string theory. I was convinced that I could fly and become pure energy and control the universe. Then I started hearing whispers. I tried again to get admitted to the hospital. This time, I licked the wall in the psychiatrist's office because I saw a dried drip mark on it and I wanted to know what it tasted like. I was told to increase one of my other medications.

My friends couldn't believe that I hadn't been admitted, and they took me to McDonald's and laid down some rules. They told me I wasn't allowed to go out on the patio alone, I shouldn't talk to strangers, and I couldn't drink alone. While they were talking, I was hugging and kissing the table because I could feel its energy and knew it was so happy and wanted to be hugged. Clearly, I was losing the capacity to judge what was appropriate.

Things got worse. I knew I was getting too sick and thought, "I'll just end this now," because I knew if I were to get well, then I'd have to deal with all the embarrassing, stupid, and irresponsible things I'd done, including some promiscuous activity, that had hurt my friends.

I got a pen and paper and was preparing to write a note, and then I was going to climb up on some scaffolding and jump off. One of my friends tried to stop me and I started to beat her with the phone—I just wanted to knock her out and put her in the closet so I could carry on with my plan. It made complete sense to me at the time.

My friends and I went to the hospital once again. In the emergency department, I told the staff that I needed to be admitted, but the psychiatrist kept asking me to explain what was going on. I cried and screamed at him, saying, "I can't explain." And then I hit him. At some level, my mind was still functioning to preserve myself, and I was desperate to get admitted or arrested so I could be put in a place where I wouldn't hurt myself or anyone else. I figured hitting the doctor would do the trick. It did.

I was in the hospital that summer for three weeks and switched to a new drug. I kept trying to tell everyone, "But I did so well on the drug and the dosage I was on at the beginning of the year. Can't that be prescribed again?" Even though I was in the hospital for three weeks, I didn't feel leveled out when I was discharged.

In July, I told my doctor that I wasn't doing well and that I was feeling overstimulated. I'm hyperaware when I'm becoming ill, and I wanted to control myself. I was trying to be responsible and get help before things got out of control. The response, once again, was to up the dosage of one of my medications to level me out. But these gradual increases didn't work. I was eventually prescribed more than the maximum dosage for this medication, and I still wasn't leveling out.

I started to lose weight. My psychiatrist presumed the weight loss was me being bulimic again and that I was the cause of my own misfortune. She wouldn't believe me when I said I thought my medication was wrong. I asked to have a different doctor, because I felt so insulted that this doctor wouldn't listen to me or give me credit for knowing myself.

My weight continued to drop. I tried to bolster my caloric intake, initially by eating healthy foods and then by eating cans and cans of icing. I eventually started drinking Ensure, but the pounds continued to fall off me. I could only fit into kids' clothing. I couldn't feel physical pain. I was so skinny and so weak that I had to drop out of school because I didn't have the strength to carry my knapsack or lift my feet high enough to get on the bus. I was so freezing cold all the time that I cried, because being so cold actually hurt.

I was also totally confused. I remember getting lost at a local shopping center. Even though this place was very familiar to me, I couldn't figure out where I was.

By September, I only weighed 103 pounds. Given that my normal weight was in the 140-pound range, I had lost 40 pounds in four months. I actually thought I was dying of cancer. I was admitted to the hospital for two weeks and was seen by an endocrinologist. I had all sorts of tests, which revealed that the huge dosage of the medication that had been gradually increased beyond its maximum dosage had overstimulated my metabolism and caused a cryothermogenic effect.

My doctor wanted to reduce this medication very quickly. This worried me, because my brain is very sensitive and I knew if I came off this drug too quickly, the effect would be to heighten all of my symptoms. I told her, "We need to do this my way, which is slowly." Her response was, "But if you want to get better, you have to follow my instructions."

Suffice it to say, my doctor and I had very different views of the appropriate road to take to achieve my well-being. She finally got fed up with me and said, "We've outgrown our relationship." That's exactly what I'd been saying to her for the past few months. I was assigned to a new doctor, a specialist in mood disorders.

Natural Allies: Partnerships in Care

At this point, this young woman, who has been sharing her story with a sense of confidence, pauses. Her lips quiver and her eyes glisten with tears. She starts to cry and apologizes. She starts to speak again, wanting to explain.

This is so hard for me to talk about, but I want to tell you what happened.

At the end of December, there was a transition meeting with my case worker, my social worker, my new psychiatrist, and my old psychiatrist. I had thought long and hard about what I wanted to say. I turned to my old psychiatrist and asked, "You've had me as a patient for three years. I'd like to know what you've learned from me throughout the course of having me as a patient, and how you will apply that knowledge in the future." Her response was, "I can't answer that."

After three years—after what I concluded were inappropriate medications and dosages and a completely wrong assessment of what my problem was, and after her thinking my weight loss was my fault—all she could say was, "I can't answer that!" I felt completely shafted. Can she really have learned nothing? Any answer would have been better than no answer. I still have no closure from this, and it really upsets me.

I am so grateful to have my new doctor. She accepts that I want to be treated as a partner in my care. She acknowledges that I'm my principal caregiver and that I'm smart enough and curious enough to figure things out. She understands that I want full clinical explanations, with proper terminology, and that I want to know about the possible side effects and interactions of medications. She is not threatened by the fact that I have my own Compendium of Pharmaceuticals and Specialties (CPS) and like looking things up. She appreciates that if I feel something is wrong, I'm usually right. She trusts that I will give her appropriate signals if I feel I'm not doing well.

I've learned so much in the past two years. I've especially learned that I need to be a collaborator in my care rather than merely a receiver of care.

Life is good now. I'm able to appreciate even the crummiest of days because there's always something wonderful to find in them.

———

Kathleen credits Laing House (www.lainghouse.org), the drop-in center, with her being alive. When her world was rudderless, it gave her a lifeline. "Kat" enjoys going to schools to talk to young men and women about her journey with mental illness. She is planning to go to college to study science.

THAT'S WHAT WE'RE HERE FOR

MY HUSBAND IS PLAGUED BY ARTHRITIS. He has had hip and knee replacements as well as operations on his back, on his shoulder, and on eight of his ten fingers. We are not strangers to the challenges of major surgery and rehabilitation. However, when Joe's second hip replacement was scheduled, we knew it would be different, because we had moved to a tiny town in the country 200 miles from the city.

Joe's surgery was going to be done in the city. However, I was going to be solely responsible for his care at home, without all the postsurgical supports of the city. I was nervous about looking after Joe. He is a big man, and I wasn't sure I would be able to move him or physically support him.

Surgery was scheduled for a Monday, and we were told that Joe would likely be discharged on Thursday. I had three days to learn what I needed to know from the nurses. I felt that if I could practice each day, I could become more comfortable and confident about taking Joe home.

When Joe was brought down to his room after surgery, the nurses asked me to leave while they got him settled. I dutifully left the room. As soon as I reached the hallway, though, I turned around and went back. I explained, "I need to be here to learn what to do." The nurses said, "No, we'll do this. That's what we're here for."

The staff could have invited me to help. In fact, my husband, a very private person, would have been more comfortable with me helping him. The nurses could have included me from the beginning. They could have taught me a little bit every day, rather than waiting until the day of discharge to tell me everything I needed to know. It's hard to process all the information you're given just before you leave.

Talking while doing doesn't take any longer, and fortunately, a couple of nurses did talk me through what they were doing and what I would need to watch for. Even with them, though, it did not feel like a partnership.

WHEN THE BRAIN IS BROKEN

"When you break your leg, your brain sends you messages that you need to do something. But when your brain is broken, those messages are scrambled or absent and you need others to be your surrogate brain. Give me a broken leg any day!"

And so began the interview with a mother of a young man in his mid-twenties who had recently experienced a second psychotic episode. She recalled events clearly, analyzed situations thoughtfully, and articulated her frustrations forcefully. This woman has been a public health nurse for years. If anyone understands health care, she does, but she is the first to admit that some things just don't make any sense.

I knew Kevin was in trouble about a week before he was to fly home for Christmas. He had told us he hadn't been feeling well, was anxious, and hadn't been sleeping. I called a friend of his and made sure someone would take him to the airport. And then I found out what I needed to know and do. For example, I called his doctor, made an appointment for Kevin for Monday morning (he was coming home on a Friday night), and asked if I could start him on the medications he had been given when he had his first psychotic episode five years earlier. And because I like to have all my bases covered, I also found out what we would have to do and say if he was really in bad shape when he arrived.

I knew right away. Kevin was escorted off the plane because he had become agitated when he tried to buy a beer during the flight and couldn't understand why the flight attendants couldn't process payment with a debit card. Then, walking down the bridge from the plane to the airport, he stopped and took off his shoes, socks, and shirt, saying that he felt really hot. By the time Kevin reached us, he was in a wheelchair, being escorted by the police. He was unkempt, and his eyes didn't look right. I knew he was psychotic.

When Kevin saw us, he said, "I just need to get home. I'm okay." But when we asked him if he had brought any luggage, he didn't know. He swung back and forth between being rational and suspicious. I knew we couldn't take him home, and so I told the police, "I'm fearful. I know he is ill. He needs to be admitted to the hospital." The police called an ambulance.

The police then explained that if Kevin did not go voluntarily and safely by ambulance, they would need to apply a section of the Mental Health Act. This would mean they would arrest him and bring him to the hospital for involuntary admission. I understood this and appreciated their caring, though difficult, description of how events might unfold.

While waiting, Kevin kept swinging in and out of control. He'd appear fine one minute and then be yelling the next. He tried to wander off, and security guards had to bring him back.

The journey to the hospital began with Kevin in the back of the ambulance and me in the front. My husband was driving our car to the hospital to meet us when we got there. Somewhere on the highway, Kevin tried to get out of the ambulance. The police were called. Kevin was arrested, put in handcuffs, and transferred to the police car to be taken to the hospital. As I moved to get into the police car, the police said I couldn't come with them. The ambulance driver piped in, saying that without a patient, he had no authority to take me. The police offered to call a taxi to take me back to the airport.

I felt like I was in the middle of a Monty Python movie! I couldn't believe what was happening—it was night, it was dark, it was December, it was cold, my husband was halfway to the city in our car with my purse, I had no money for a taxi and no car at the airport, and our son was in a full-blown psychotic state with handcuffs around his wrists! I burst into tears, which was completely unlike me. Eventually, the ambulance driver figured out how to bend the rules to take me to the hospital.

At the hospital, Kevin was triaged right into psychiatry. I asked Kevin if he wanted me to be with him, and he said yes. He admitted to seeing things and hearing voices. The psychiatrist asked me if anything like this had happened before—*yes, five years ago*—what the previous diagnosis had been—*acute mania with psychosis*—and if he was on medication—*no, he had been taken off his antipsychotic medication by his psychiatrist three months after his first episode.* And then she asked Kevin if he had taken any drugs—*I smoked some dope*—if he was hearing voices or seeing things—*yes (as he was slowly trying to wipe something invisible to me off the walls)*—and if he was feeling violent—*no (but the psychiatrist had seen him earlier when Kevin had been much more agitated)*. She finally concluded, "Yes, we need to give him some oral medication and admit him." You cannot imagine my relief.

Kevin was transferred to the mental health hospital and put in protective isolation. We went home at 2:30 in the wee hours of the morning. The very next day, we had our first taste of being cut out of the loop of information.

Overnight, we went from being the parents who'd been through this before, who'd been part of Kevin's recovery before, and who were able to provide background information relevant to the situation (like triggers, details of the first admission, diagnosis, and what medication he'd been on after the first psychotic episode) to being parents who would be told nothing because the patient was an adult fully protected by the system's "protection of privacy." Even for simple questions like, "How did Kevin sleep last night?" all we'd get back was, "You'll have to ask him; we cannot tell you."

Over time, I learned who might give me scraps of information and who would hold hard and fast to the privacy rules. Typically it was nurses with more experience and a higher comfort level who showed some compassion toward us. It was still like a bit of a game, though. For example, rather than asking directly about how Kevin had slept, I had learned to carefully pick a "good" nurse and say, "Kevin says he slept well last night." And then I'd get back, "Well, we have a different definition of 'well,' because he actually walked the halls all night."

As time progressed, Kevin was given passes to come home to stay with us on weekends. He was having his medications changed based on his symptoms and side effects, but we were never told what the medications were now. At the most, we might get something like, "We've increased his meds because he's still showing symptoms."

We learned that if we weren't going to be given information, then we would at least provide the hospital staff with observations we had. For example, we might say, "Kevin had a good weekend, but he still doesn't seem to think this is a chronic condition that he'll have to manage for some time." We figured out that the more we talked to the nurses about things when there wasn't a crisis, the more they were willing to share with us. Sometimes I would find myself feeling clever when we'd get a scrap of information, and then I'd remind myself that this whole situation was ridiculous.

When Kevin was being discharged, I asked his psychiatrist, "Do you have a diagnosis?" He replied, "I can't share that with you without Kevin's permission." I tried to make sense of this: His brain is broken, yet he is the only one who can give the professionals permission to talk to us and provide information about his care? I wanted to scream!

Instead I said, "Okay—help me understand this. In the emergency room, it was important that I knew what his diagnosis had been from before and what medications he'd been on. And if I hadn't known, we would have all been flying blind, because it took five days for his previous records to be faxed from 3,000 miles away and they were illegible when they arrived anyway."

All the literature says (of course I'd been reading up on this) that the more stable, supportive, and enriching environment you can give someone who has had a psychotic episode, as well as the shorter the time a person is in psychosis, the better the recovery. Yet basic information was being withheld from us. What was I supposed to say if we had to take Kevin back to emergency one day? "Oh, I'm so sorry, we aren't allowed to know—you'll have to ask the person who is trying to wipe imaginary objects off the wall!"

We signed up for a nine-week course for families of youth with early psychosis, and this helped a lot. For starters, we discovered that everyone was similarly frustrated by the lack of sharing of information. It also opened up a lot of doors with Kevin. For example, we might say to him, "We heard last night that some families have worked out a relapse plan with their son or daughter." And he might reply, "Yeah—that has come up in my education sessions as well. I guess we should talk about it some time."

Weeks passed and Kevin improved. He was able to live with us and be supported during his recovery. Someone else in his situation, without a family with the means to provide love and financial support, would have been on the street, homeless.

We know that with each episode of psychosis, the person's recovery takes longer and is less complete. The idea, therefore, is to try to prevent reoccurrences. As Kevin's parents, we want to try to catch symptoms early and prevent another full-blown episode. I just wish we had more information to help us. We are relatively lucky—at least Kevin is open to telling us, when asked, about his medication dosages. His diagnosis? The "provisional" diagnosis remained: psychosis NOS (not otherwise specified). This is what the nurses told me I could say if required in the future.

If I had to rate the people we dealt with through all this on a scale of 10, 10 being the highest, I'd give 9.5 to the police; 9 to the ambulance staff; 8.5 to the emergency room staff; 9 to the psychiatrist we saw in emergency; somewhere between 7 and 8 for the nurses at the mental health hospital; only a 1 or 2 to the in-patient psychiatrist at that hospital; similarly, only a 1 or 2 to the discharge planning process; and a 7 or 8 to the outpatient services.

By comparison, I'd walk over broken glass for the psychiatrist we had in the remote community we'd lived in before, the first time Kevin got sick and his dad had to bring him home from college in France. That doctor's focus was community mental health. He knew we were there for Kevin and instrumental to his recovery. He told us everything and supported all of us through every step along the road of Kevin's recovery.

We move forward by inches. We watch everything for signs of relapse. We pick our words carefully before we say something, because we want to keep the doors of communication and trust open with Kevin. Situations like this change everything about your life and your relationships.

There are gifts as well as pain. I feel I've become more empathetic. It has even changed how I read the newspaper. I now think that maybe some of the people who are reported as having done bad things are really people suffering from mental health problems.

When the Brain Is Broken

It's so ironic that everyone talks about the importance of taking the secretiveness and stigma out of mental illness, and yet our experience was that information was and still is hidden from us. Mental illness is treated differently from a privacy perspective. When my husband had knee surgery, the doctors and nurses told me everything without asking his permission. There's a double standard.

There needs to be a better balance between protection of an individual's privacy and involving the family so that they can provide the most informed support possible. The challenges we experienced in the name of "protection of privacy" need to be addressed and better handled. The overriding spirit and intention must be to provide the best possible care for someone. After all, we both want the same health outcome—a fully functioning member of our family and society.

At this point, this mother stops talking. She is obviously hesitating, thinking about what to say next. And then she lowers her voice and says, "I wasn't too sure about talking to you today. But then I asked myself if I wanted to be the kind of person I might otherwise criticize for not speaking out. There's so much to do about the stigma around mental health. But you know, I still wonder if I'll say anything in our Christmas letter this year about what happened to Kevin. I know if he'd broken his leg, I'd mention it. But to say he had a psychotic episode . . . I just don't know."

At the time of writing, eleven months had passed since that frightening December. Kevin was doing well and living on his own and holding down a professional job that he loves.

IT TAKES A TEAM

APPEARANCES CAN SOMETIMES BE DECEIVING. Picture a young couple, relaxing and playing with their healthy and happy four-month-old son before they have dinner. This delightful image, frozen as a single snapshot, shows neither the months of agony and panic that preceded this evening nor the many people who played important roles in getting to this moment in time. Where to begin?

"What was the most touching thing that happened to you when Jakob was born?" The dad doesn't hesitate and says, "The taxi driver!" His wife nods in agreement and tears spring to their eyes.

The dad explains. "It was two days after Jakob's birth and death. We were leaving the hospital and got in a taxi for the short ride home. I told the driver we had just lost our son, so would he mind turning the music down? We drove in silence. When we got home, my wife went inside right away. The taxi driver got out of his car, came up to me, put his hand on my shoulder, and said, 'We lost a daughter.' He was a complete stranger, but I'll never forget him. You might wonder what were the odds of us taking that taxi with that driver. But I find that every time we turn around, we hear about stillborn babies."

Shannon's pregnancy had been miserable: nausea beyond belief, continuous bleeding, and occasional high blood pressure. Regular testing, though, showed everything to be proceeding appropriately.

She picks up the story.

I went into labor at 6 A.M. on July 12, 2004. We called the hospital, and the folks there said to come in and be checked. When we arrived, we were admitted to the assessment unit, and a nurse named Judy was assigned to us. She checked for the baby's heartbeat but couldn't find it right away. She tried to reassure us by saying, "Oh, he's probably just moving around right now— I'll keep trying." She tried several times. We started to panic, and I broke down.

Judy took us into another room, where she told us they'd do an ultrasound. She began to gently prepare us by saying, "It will be good to check, but I think we would have found it by now." After the ultrasound, a doctor confirmed our worst fears and said, "Yup! He's gone." Apparently this man is a genius and is the one called in for the most complicated obstetrical cases. He must see tragedy every day and has even lost a child of his own, but he seemed almost cavalier or nonchalant as he told us that our son, Jakob, was dead. Maybe that's how he copes.

Of course, my labor had to continue and play itself out. It took sixteen hours. My grief was like a drug. I felt like I was seeing and hearing everything under water.

The dad speaks again.

While Shannon was still in labor, a social worker came in. I hated her the first time I met her. She came in to offer support but then asked about arrangements for the body and had me start to fill out paperwork for the death certificate. I almost yelled at her, because I didn't want to see anyone, let alone talk about details of the death of our baby, who hadn't even been born yet! Couldn't she have waited until the next day? Couldn't she have filled out the paperwork herself and just have me sign?

I have to say, I didn't ever want to see this woman again. However, she got a second chance, and ultimately, she was very helpful and an important support for us. For example, after we went home, she stayed in touch with us by calling every week or two. She also recommended someone for me to talk to. And when we became pregnant with Noah, she helped us get used to visiting the hospital and becoming comfortable being there without freaking out.

The person the social worker suggested I talk to was the hospital chaplain, a priest. I thought this was an odd choice, because I am not religious in any conventional way. I've never talked to a priest who hasn't tried to push something on me. But this man was a million times more a therapist than the therapist I ended up with. He was a decent and good person, and I appreciated his honesty. I remember asking him, "What do you tell people who ask how can God do this?" He said, "I hope they don't ask."

Then Shannon pipes in.

Of course, we got to see Jakob that night, but not for long. But I do wish we could have seen him again, a second time, the next day. I also wish someone had suggested that we take a camera to the funeral home so that we could have had a picture of him there. The hospital gave us a beautiful memory box with Jakob's official certificates, a lock of his hair, a picture taken of him after I delivered him, his handprints and footprints, and the clothing he wore. We treasure this.

The nurse assigned to us when we arrived at the hospital that morning stayed with us long after her shift ended. She also came up to see us the next morning before her shift started. She stayed for half an hour. We talked and cried. I can't tell you one word that was said, but the fact that she took time out of her day to acknowledge our experience will stay with me as a warm memory forever.

The next morning, we were exhausted and in a daze. There were two nurses who were great with us. They seemed to be moving at a hyper-efficient speed but were very kind. For example, they urged Sean to get in bed with me and snuggle; we didn't know we could do that.

The dad now wants to make a point. "Nurses are fantastic. The way we see it, they do all the work. They bring you the ice chips, they rub your shoulders, and they're there for you as people. They treat you as the most important people in the world and form a relationship with you. Nurses seem willing to share themselves with you, while doctors don't."

His voice drops and his tone softens.

Time at home was hard. We had expected to come home with a baby, but our baby was dead. When a baby is stillborn, you don't even have memories. I remember that the night before he was born, I shone the flashlight at Shannon's stomach. Everywhere the light fell, Jakob would kick that spot. It was the only time I ever got to play with him.

When I went back to work, everyone asked how Shannon was doing, but nobody asked about me. Dads get left out of the loop. In our society, guys are supposed to be tough. I guess I was anything but tough, because seven months later, I crashed. I hadn't slept for a week; I kept having the same images when I closed my eyes. I was working as hard and as much as I could, but I kept my door closed because I'd cry a lot. I'd never felt that bad in my life, and I expected that I should have been feeling better. After all, more than six months had passed and, in theory, things were looking up. I liked my job, we'd been on a vacation, and Shannon was pregnant again. But I was in a constant state of panic and couldn't handle anything.

I think the new pregnancy terrified me. It's not like there was any point in time we could relax and feel confident. For example, if people have had a miscarriage at ten weeks, then they feel somewhat confident that things will be okay when the pregnancy reaches twelve or fourteen weeks. For us, our panic increased as time passed, because our worst point of reference was the last point of reference.

Fortunately, ever since Jakob died, we'd been seeing our family doctor once a week, just to talk. She could see what was happening. She read me the riot act and said I had to take time off of work. She wanted me to take two months off—we compromised on one. She also gave me some structure, some things I had to do: I had to eat well, get daily exercise, and leave the house every day. I spent a lot of time bawling in a park I found. I just let it all hang out.

When asked what helped them with their grief and their fears around the second pregnancy, they answer together:

A bunch of things, really. First of all, Noah was a very active baby and moved at thirteen weeks, so that helped. Also, the fact that we could see our family doctor every week and that everyone in her office was so welcoming and kind and understanding gave us regular support we cherished. We also rented a Doppler machine so we could test for the baby's heartbeat when we were stressing out. Our family doctor helped us not let this become an obsession and get out of control. She told us to use the machine only twice a day, and then only once a day, and then to go a couple of days without using it.

We also hooked up with an Internet web site for people who had lost a child. It was comforting to not have to explain ourselves to any of these people. They knew. We knew. And they had tips and coping strategies that were so helpful to us. We could even offer advice to others based on our experiences.

Shannon provides more details about the support they received.

I was able to connect with a couple of mothers locally who had had a stillborn child. Sometimes I just needed to talk to someone who would listen and who understood what I was talking about. Another woman I knew from work had a child who died when she was five years old. This woman sent me a Mother's Day card that May. She understood that we were still mothers.

During the second pregnancy, we had fabulous attention and care. We had ultrasounds once a month and were checked once a week for planning scores. We were given every assessment and indication possible that this baby seemed lively and fine. But as we got closer to the end of the pregnancy, we became terrified. At thirty-seven weeks, we'd had it. We couldn't stand the stress and asked to be induced. We were prepared with a speech about how we wouldn't leave the doctor's office, but we didn't have to give the speech. The doctor understood what we were going through. He said he'd do a test to make sure the baby's lungs were mature and, if so, we'd be good to go!

I was induced at thirty-seven weeks. The contractions were four minutes apart and the labor went on, seemingly forever. After twenty-nine hours, the fetal heart rate dropped from 160 to 80. Within thirty seconds, we went from having just a single nurse in our room to having a doctor, a resident, some medical students, and several nurses. The intensity was palpable as I was told, "This baby is going to be born in the next five minutes or we're going to do a cesarean section." You cannot imagine our fear.

Within five minutes, Noah was born, and he cried right away. Our family doctor had tears pouring down her face. In fact, I think everyone in the room was crying. Finally, we experienced pure joy after a day full of panic.

When you come home with a new baby, you suddenly think, "What do I do with him?" We now have a new person to add to our list of heroes! The public health nurse has saved our sanity more than once. She helped me through my breasts becoming engorged; she determined that Noah had a hernia and needed surgery (successful); she just drops in to say hi; and she recommended a nearby family resource center. We go to the family resource center regularly, and there's another public health nurse who comes to that center every Wednesday. I always know there's someone I can easily check in with for reassurance.

Amidst all these shared memories, Sean and Shannon hardly ever take their eyes off Noah. These three are each delightful and are clearly delighting in each other. But they are the first to say they didn't get to this point in time alone. They give testimony to the fact that it takes a team to support grief, to nurture a pregnancy, and to reinforce the early days, weeks, and months of becoming a family.

INVESTING IN INFORMATION

THE RECOVERY ROOM NURSES ALWAYS TOLD ME THAT MY MAXILLO-FACIAL SURGERY PATIENTS WERE EASY TO MANAGE POSTOPERATIVELY. They said they could tell that my patients were well prepared. I appreciated their positive comments. I don't mean to sound like I'm blowing my own horn, but recovery room nurses know their stuff. They can even tell you what level of anxiety a patient had been feeling when being anesthetized.

I knew a nurse who had jaw reconstruction and who understood what it was like to have her jaw wired closed. I would always try to get her to talk to my patients before they went in for surgery. I would also tell my patients, when they were coming to see me, to write down their questions. I told them, "You might be nervous and forget to ask me what's on your mind."

And in the evenings, I would call every patient I'd operated on that day to see how they were doing. These calls tended to confirm my hunch that people are usually uptight when they're coming in for surgery, even if it's only day surgery, and they aren't always paying attention, even to written postoperative instructions.

I started making these calls for a selfish reason: I was practicing by myself and I didn't particularly want to get called at midnight. Adding an hour of phone calls to the end of my workday gave me my nights and addressed patients' concerns before they became serious problems.

All the problems I'd seen in my years of becoming a surgeon boiled down to communication issues. I just talked to my patients the way I'd like someone to talk to me.

IT JUST COMES NATURALLY

*Dr. Ann-Marie Thomas is Director of Inpatient Physical
Medicine and Rehabilitation Services and Medical Director
of Neuromuscular Rehabilitation at Spaulding Rehabilitation
Hospital. She is also an Instructor at the Harvard Medical
School. In 2001, Dr. Thomas was given the Compassionate
Caregiver Award by the Kenneth B. Schwartz Center.*

WHEN ASKED WHAT IT FELT LIKE TO BE SINGLED OUT FOR THE
COMPASSIONATE CAREGIVER AWARD, Dr. Ann-Marie Thomas said,
"The hardest part about getting this award is that what I consider everyday care is what others think makes me stand out. I don't
think what I do is special."

When pressed, Dr. Thomas admits that she can see some differences between the way she practices medicine and what others do. She quickly adds that she would prefer not to stand out;
that she would prefer others to do what she does. Dr. Thomas
believes that the way she practices medicine is simply common
sense. She adds, "It also gets the best results for my patients."

Dr. Thomas elaborates on four elements of her approach,
which she says "just comes naturally":

**I actually spend enough time with patients to get to know
them.** Nobody is just their medical problem. When somebody
presents with a sore shoulder, I need to find out about that
patient's whole life. I've found that the more you invest in the
relationship with a patient, the more you'll get back. They open
up and tell you everything. I learn things that affect my decisions
about treatment and care.

I'm stunned that doctors can see patients so quickly. They just fly in and out. When I went to see a doctor recently, I had my mouth open to ask a question, but he was already gone. I made another appointment and when he came in, before he could open his mouth, I said, "I'm just here to talk."

My patient is the patient *and* his or her extended family. This view is especially important in my world of rehabilitative medicine, where problems are often complicated, chronic or progressive, and emotionally challenging. I recall a particular patient who was a retired neurologist with a debilitating brain disorder. He had deteriorated to the point where he could no longer be managed at home. I spent a huge amount of time with this man's wife, helping her contact and consult with family, listening to her host of worries, and comforting her through the decisions she had to make. When she first approached me, it was a busy day, and so I suggested, "I only have five minutes right now, but let's use our time together to figure out when we can get together for half an hour." I put her on my schedule later that day.

I'm a big advocate for having an educated patient, and, if the patient can't learn, then I make sure I educate someone else in the family. I want my patients to become partners in their care. To do that, they have to know everything—what they have, what's being done, why it's being done, what their medications are, what side effects to watch for, and what to expect and ask for when they go to see other doctors. The returns on this are huge. Patients are more compliant with their medications and treatments. If I'm away, even though I leave complete and exhaustive notes, the patient helps educate the doctor filling in for me.

It Just Comes Naturally

It is important to empower people at the beginning of the relationship. I give patients and families my e-mail address so they can send me their questions and concerns. They also know they can call me if they are in a bind.

My work often combines elements of physical rehabilitation with addictions counseling. I recall one man who came to us because he had to have a limb amputated and because of his forty-five-year-long alcohol addiction. This man had been in hundreds of detox programs before he came to us, but none had worked for him. We were going to have to manage his withdrawal from alcohol postoperatively.

I got to know this man very well. I found out he had twelve children, all of whom had cut him off because of his alcoholism. I came to understand how desperately he wanted to reconnect with his family. I committed to work with him. Even when he was discharged, I would call him at home just to check in. If he missed an appointment, I'd call to ask if something was wrong. And he called me, not only when he was troubled, fearing a relapse, but also when he was overjoyed, having been invited to a family function.

Because I had also coached him on what to look for and what to ask for if he had to go to a doctor in his community, one day he called me from the emergency room. He knew something was wrong, but the hospital wanted to send him home. He was trying to advocate for himself but needed help. I spoke to the doctors and told them what tests he needed. The tests showed that he had clots in his leg and lung. Had he gone home, he could well have been dead in an hour.

This patient wrote about Dr. Thomas. "There was something missing (in the detox programs I'd been in). I don't know what it was. Dr. Thomas took me—a weak, trembling, confused, and very fearful individual—out of a wheelchair and gave me the gift of inspiration. She talked to me whenever and for whatever time I needed, busy as she was! She listened and helped me understand the disease of addiction. She is reassuring and compassionate and has exceeded any medical treatment and attention I have ever experienced in my seventy-two years."

I always try to be patient and to imagine being in my patients' shoes. Another example illustrates what I mean by this. I had a patient who, until she became incapacitated by ALS, also known as Lou Gehrig's disease, had been a computer programmer for the Pentagon. Her mind was completely intact, but she had lost her ability to speak. She was still able to communicate, though, with a letter board and on the computer.

Many staff would not take the time to "listen" while she painstakingly tried to say what was on her mind. One day, the nurses were trying to wash her, and she kept saying "no." The staff were horrified and complained to me that she didn't care about being cleaned. Of course, I asked her what had happened. It turned out that she was saying "no" because she desperately needed suctioning. The staff hadn't taken the time to figure out that she was making an appropriate choice between her priority of being able to breathe and their priority of her being clean.

I told the nurses that "not communicating is not an option. We have to own this problem and figure it out." Working with the patient, we ended up coming up with a list of common requests she might have and creating a communication board for the nurses. Now, this woman doesn't have to take a long time to communicate her basic wishes. Now, it's simple and quick. All she has to do is point her head to a spot on the list. At first the nurses were resistant to working with this woman, but now they are seeing the benefits of solving the problem. The patient has taken time to praise them for their efforts.

It takes time to work with staff and to sensitize them to patients' points of view, but the returns are so easy to see. For example, some medical students and interns were just barging into patients' rooms as though the rooms were extensions of the hallway. I explained that the patients' rooms are, in fact, like their homes while they are with us. "Would you barge into someone's house without knocking?" I asked. That's all it took. Now they knock.

I love working with medical students. I just hope that what they learn with me sticks. I want them to know that I continue to be amazed by the power of the patient-caregiver relationship. I want them to know that I have learned that a big hug can be as therapeutic as an antibiotic, a smile as comforting as an analgesic, and a kind word or hand on the shoulder more uplifting than any medical procedure.

It's about being human. As doctors, we should not be on any pedestal—we should be partners in an equal relationship. I hope my passion for my work and for the patients and families I serve is contagious.

My ten-year-old says he was born to be a football player. Well, I was born to be a doctor. I wanted to be a doctor from the time I was four and was playing doctor with dolls and delivering their babies long before I actually knew where they came from. My parents tried to discourage me. I even tried to discourage myself when I found out how long it would take to become a doctor. But being a doctor is all I've ever wanted to be. Taking care of someone's health is more of a privilege than anything else I can think of. It's almost sacred.

AWASH IN DISAPPOINTMENT

The following letter was written by a mother, Donna, in the middle of a Sunday night, after more than two weeks of waiting and watching. The letter was a plea to a doctor that her daughter, Jane, had seen a year earlier. The mother wrote to this particular doctor because he was familiar with her daughter, the cystic fibrosis team, and the team system. Perhaps even more importantly, this doctor was someone the family felt had liked and admired their daughter's determination to recover from an infection in her blood that he'd never seen anyone recover from before. This doctor had said that it had been "a privilege to be part of the miracle of her recovery" the year before.

At the time of the writing of this letter, Donna's daughter, Jane, was in her mid twenties. Jane had been diagnosed with cystic fibrosis at four months of age. Donna's older son had also had cystic fibrosis and had died five and a half years earlier.

DEAR DR.__: This is what I have watched over the last three weeks.

Wednesday, May 21

Jane arrives home from Circus School and goes directly to the freezer for ice. Okay—a rib issue—could it be another stress fracture—or maybe it's just a muscle. The ice was applied—the modest pain numbed—maybe it's a muscle. It's over a year and a half since the last stress fracture, and we know what happened after that . . . the DISASTROUS hospital stay. Let's hope it's just muscle.

Awash in Disappointment

Sunday, May 25

Jane is on the sofa and pale. Yes, it's the rib—full out and full pain. Okay, then off to bed for full rest—see if we can't rest this into relief from the pain. Try lots of ibuprofen for inflammation and pain relief. Just stay in bed to allow it to heal. Oh, and how about we do two extra masks and extra sessions of physio every day from now on. Let's keep this from getting out of hand.

Tuesday, May 27

No one has to be this miserable—let's get something for the pain. Total fatigue—touch of fever—pure exhaustion from fighting the pain. Oh, and a prescription for antibiotics, too. Let's be really safe and go back on those—after just three days, off of them. Coughing is hard with a sore rib. All the extra care we can have, that we need, so this doesn't get out of hand.

A call to the cystic fibrosis nurse coordinator for advice. The head doctor is out of town. A call to another doctor who prescribes Tylenol with codeine. I go to pick it up—oh, it's not there. Prescriptions like that need to be picked up at the doctor's office to take to the dispensary. We didn't know that. So off to the office and then back to the dispensary—paper in hand—to get the pills. Lucky I'd told Jane I'd go pick them up—she would have collapsed in pain with all the going back and forth.

Wednesday, May 28

Pain pills helped for sleeping and resting. With the rest and the physio and masks, maybe the cough will stay under control. Let's be patient and the healing should be starting.

Thursday, May 29

Out of bed and off to the airport at supper time to pick up Jane's friend from Boston. Taking it slowly—a nice distraction from the hard week of pain and fatigue.

Friday, May 30

A slow approach to the day—a walk in the park—and out for dinner. Pain can be lived with—but oh so tired. Tylenol with codeine will do that. But lots of masks and physio should help keep that cough from sneaking up.

Saturday, May 31

Sore, but not as bad—but so tired and short of breath . . . really short of breath. So short of breath that a walk up the stairs is trouble. One block up the street is trouble. Damn. It seems we're in trouble. Those extra masks are some relief. The physio should be helping. This is June—asthma time of year—could it be that? The cough isn't that bad, but the shortness of breath—not good. Jane thinks prednisone should help. Let's just start with a few days at fifty milligrams and see. That should help ease the shortness of breath.

Sunday, June 1

A day of worry and wait. Maybe the breathing will be better tomorrow. Those extra masks, physio—not so much pain now. That rib must be healing. No fevers, not too full a chest—it must be allergies. Surely the prednisone will kick in and ease that shortness of breath.

Awash in Disappointment

Monday, June 2

Okay, we'll watch this puffing, shortness of breath, breathing coming and going—we should get something. This is hard to watch.

Tuesday, June 3

I can't take it anymore. I call the nurse coordinator myself. My thoughts—an IV solumedrol. They did that on one admission, and Jane thought it was the most effective treatment. Maybe we could try that? Could it be done as an outpatient? In emergency? Let's get some relief for this shortness of breath.

Wednesday, June 4

The nurse coordinator says, "Before we prescribe we want to assess, so send Jane over for a pulmonary function test, blood test, and an X-ray." Great! This is all done before noon. We'll get some answers, some treatment, and some relief from the shortness of breath and the cough that is creeping up and getting a bit worse. The head doctor won't be seeing Jane—but will let us know the course of action after the results are in. Wonder if that solumedrol would just ease the situation? Or do we need IV antibiotics now, too? No calls by the end of the day . . . as we wait.

Thursday, June 5

Okay, it's 2:30 in the afternoon and no calls yet. What does this mean? I'm calling to find out. Oh . . . the head doctor won't be there all day but will call on Friday. Okay, we'll sit here, waiting, watching Jane in her discomfort—short of breath and with a cough that's getting worse. We'll do the extra masks and physio, and we'll try to think that something can be done here to keep us out of the hospital . . . because we know where that went last time. But what has to be, has to be. They'll be in at 8 A.M. and so we'll just wait.

Friday, June 6

Are those flushed cheeks from the high dosage of steroids? Is that a slight fever? When will they call? What are we doing here? It's Friday—it's too late to do anything.

Okay, it's 2:30 in the afternoon—I'm calling again. I ask the nurse coordinator, "What's up? What's the plan?" She says, "Oh, we're just finishing clinic. We'll call you back shortly."

At 3:30, she calls. "Okay, the plan—home IV antibiotics for two weeks. It's Friday, so we'll start it all on Monday. Pic line in at noon, pick up meds in the afternoon. A run-through with the home IV people. The X-rays don't look too bad. If it were asthma, the steroids would have helped but haven't. Switch to medrol from prednisone."

What's that, I wonder, and why—and why not IV steroids? With all the planning for Monday, I forget to ask.

Saturday, June 7

Not such a great day—a bit achy, a hint of fever at the start of the day. But after all, we'll be on meds by Monday night. I see a thermometer on the counter. Has she been worrying about her fever? Is she not telling us, not wanting us to worry? It's a Saturday, so there's no point in talking about fevers. There's nothing that's going to be done until late Monday.

Awash in Disappointment

Sunday, June 8

It sure is hard to watch someone so short of breath. It sure is hard to hear someone cough that hard. It sure is hard not to be worried totally to a frazzle as you wait for it to be Monday. It sure is hard to have to be saying, "Sure, I think two weeks of home IV will do the job, dear."

The point is that *it is all hard*. So, here are my questions:

1. Why seven days—from Tuesday to Monday—before any single change to my daughter's treatment takes place?

2. Would it not have been appropriate for someone—a doctor—to actually see Jane? Or is she just the sum of her blood test, X-rays, and pulmonary function tests?

3. Would a doctor, seeing her shortness of breath, not have recognized the need for relief for her?

4. Don't we all know that nothing happens on weekends? But illness and symptoms don't take weekends off.

5. Can you imagine the emotional toll here for our family, for these last days? Watching, rationalizing, worrying, quietly praying, pretending.

This has been long and rambling, I know.

What would I have wanted? That I call a doctor on a Tuesday and someone sees my daughter, recognizes a situation, and moves on it.

But what have I seen? That I call a doctor on Tuesday, and it's now the middle of the night on Sunday, and we're no further ahead. But how much ground did we lose while waiting?

The most important thought—"Where's the preventative approach to cystic fibrosis treatment?"

For more than twenty years we have approached this disease with, "How do we prevent problems?" But for the past eight years—and let's say it—under the umbrella of adult care—the approach has been, "How do we treat problems?"

The distinction is crucial. A seven-day delay prevents nothing. A seven-day delay provides lots of problems to treat.

How do we work to change this?

Can you and I have a chat to talk about it?

I ask this of you because of who and what you are and who you have been for us.

Help us make this work better. We need to for Jane, and we need to for all the others.

—Donna

Five weeks later, on Tuesday, July 15, Jane died.

Now, two and a half years later, Donna says that she is not awash in bitterness that her two children had cystic fibrosis and have now died. She says that she is awash in disappointment and frustration that she hasn't been able to make the world of adult care better for others with cystic fibrosis.

Donna, along with her husband and her children, knew the world of cystic fibrosis and hospitals intimately. She explains that their experiences within the world of pediatrics had shown them all what the gold standard of care can be. In pediatrics, their experience was that the care of children with cystic fibrosis was focused on the potential for full lives, on problem prevention, and on involving and respecting patients and families. She even recalls, with some fondness, the day they learned that their son also had cystic fibrosis. She had called the doctor's office to find out if the results were in and was told that the doctor would call her right back. The next thing she knew was that the pediatrician was at the door of her house. He said, "I couldn't give you this news over the phone."

Both of Jane's parents had been very involved in local, national, and international organizations devoted to cystic fibrosis. In spite of their demonstrated deep commitment to the field and their intimate knowledge about the care of their children, Donna says that when her children moved from the world of pediatrics to the world of adult care, she felt she was labeled as aggressive, intrusive, overprotective, pampered, and spoiled. Donna asks:

Does expecting the best care for my children make me spoiled? Does knowing that a high standard of care existed one block away make me pampered? What is aggressive about asking for the same level of care in the world of adult medicine?

As a family, we had always put our thoughts together to see what we could be doing as a game plan, what we might want to talk over with the doctors, what questions we would have, what advice we were looking for. In the adult hospital, we never felt that the staff were partners with us. We felt we had to be the ones to know about treatment options and what needed to be done. We felt we had to know everything, to ask for everything, to start at the very beginning with every new person. They didn't seem to care, and they conveyed an attitude of, "Well, your child has cystic fibrosis—he or she is going to die."

The so-called "team" was fragmented, and they never pulled together. You never knew who you'd see, because the doctors in the clinic and on the wards changed every month or two. The senior doctor, who was the one constant person, rarely came to see our children, even when they were admitted. If the person at the top of the chain isn't in the room checking on patients, what's a resident to do?

Very early on, in the adult hospital world, my husband and I asked for a meeting with one of the hospital vice-presidents. We wanted to make a case for some of the difficulties we were having; to share some of what we'd learned from our children's years under pediatric care and also from our wide involvement in the world of cystic fibrosis organizations; and to offer our help to improve the situation, not only for our own children, but also generally. But all the vice-president could talk about was "process" and "the system" and "the needs of the hospital." He had no concept of patient- or family-centered care.

I tried every avenue I could think of. I even went to the hospital's ombudsman. He listened with great empathy and admitted that he was powerless to bring about any change. I went through the social work department. I offered to help the cystic fibrosis nurse coordinator, explaining that my role was not to criticize but to be an advocate for the nurses and the important work they do. No one ever picked up on any offers of help.

No one can accuse me of having vested interests now, and I'd still like to help bring about changes to make the adult care of people with cystic fibrosis better. But I can't tell you how powerless I felt. I saw so many changes that were desperately needed, yet I was not able to make a difference. It is a source of deep despair for me.

~

More Than Words:
Feeling Heard and Being Valued

"It is ironic that awareness, intentionality, and kindness
may still be sadly undernourished in many
hospital settings, especially since these qualities
are what hospitals are ostensibly all about.
The very word 'hospital' betokens 'hospitality',
an honored greeting, a true receiving.
But somehow it is still all too easy within hospitals
and the stream of medical care, although nobody
intends for it to happen, to get lost, to not
be met or heard or fully seen, and to not be followed
to the point of completion and personal satisfaction."
—*Jon Kabat-Zinn*

"To laugh often and much; to win the respect of
intelligent people and the affection of children . . . to leave
the world a better place . . . to know even one life has
breathed easier because of you. This is to have succeeded."
—*Ralph Waldo Emerson*

~

What is the message contained in a greeting of genuine warmth? How important is a phone call to just "check in?" If I am referred to as my disease or symptom, do I disappear as a person? If someone asks about my life, apart from my illness, does that mean I am whole?

It is truly amazing what people remember from health care experiences. While medical science can do so much to treat and heal people, it is often the human touches that matter so much and are remembered for years: being called by name, a gentle touch on a shoulder, the timely sharing of anxiously awaited information, the extra time taken for all the questions in the world, comparing pictures of children, discussing books read or movies seen.

A TRIPLE WIN
SURGICAL SUSPENSE ON SUNDAYS
THE HEALING EFFECT OF LISTENING
TATTOO IT ON OUR HEARTS
AN ENORMOUS BURDEN IS LIFTED
WHERE'S THE HEADACHE?
I'M THE FULL-TIME TENANT OF THIS BODY
THE VALUE OF ASKING QUESTIONS

A TRIPLE WIN

IT WAS A CRAZY TIME. My mother was in one hospital, having had a stroke at age ninety-three. My niece was in another hospital, having given birth to premature twins. And my 101-year-old father-in-law was in a third hospital. Like a hamster on a wheel, I just kept going around in circles, visiting everyone.

And then came the day when it was decided that my niece and the twins would be discharged. In another hospital across the city, a similar decision was being reached about my mother. She was going to be discharged the very same day.

My only sister was an ocean and a continent away. It was up to me to get my mother and my niece and her twins settled into their homes. Everyone was anxious about going home, but no one was admitting it.

I got my niece and the babies settled in first and told them I'd be back. And then I took my mother to her home, a high-rise apartment building for seniors, where she proudly lived independently. I was afraid about leaving her alone—afraid she'd fall—but I had to keep moving.

I quickly went home to get something, and that was when I got a call saying my father-in-law had died. But I had to keep moving.

I made a phone call to check in on my niece. She said that the babies were sleeping and that she was okay. Then phone calls to tell relatives about my father-in-law and more phone calls to begin to plan a funeral. Finally, I called my mother, who replied, uncharacteristically, when I asked how she was doing, "Not too good, dear."

Shortly after this, a nurse from the unit my mother had been on called from the hospital just to see how Mum was doing. I think I burst into tears. I told her I was worried about Mum and also told her that my father-in-law had just died a couple of hours earlier.

Later that night, my mother's doctor called from the unit. He said, "I understand there's a lot going on in your life right now. You know, I've been thinking. We haven't actually completed the discharge papers for your mother, and so we think it's best if you just bring her back in. We'll take care of her at least until the funeral is over. We'll also do another assessment before we send her home again. We know that when someone has a stroke, we're dealing with the whole family." Amazing! He actually said that.

And so I took Mum back to the hospital. She was relieved, because she really wasn't ready to be home. She stayed for another two weeks, and the investment of that extra time enabled her to live on her own for another four years. I'll never forget that doctor's compassion. His decision ended up being good for her, good for me, and good for the health care system.

SURGICAL SUSPENSE ON SUNDAYS

MY MOTHER-IN-LAW'S HEALTH HAD BEEN FAILING AT HOME. She was admitted to the hospital to try to determine what was going on. After a week in the hospital, she was having trouble breathing. It was decided to do exploratory surgery. The situation seemed very serious, and the family was notified. My mother-in-law was given Last Rites on Sunday morning, and the operation was scheduled to start at 1:00 P.M.

The family was taken to a waiting room. Time passed. No one came out to tell us anything. By 6:30 P.M., I said that I would try to find out what was going on if we still hadn't heard anything by 7:00 P.M. But I could only wait another fifteen minutes—I was desperate for some information.

My sister-in-law came with me. The first problem we had was that we couldn't find anyone to ask. No one was anywhere to be found. We finally found a nurse who directed us to a phone with a direct line into the operating room suite. A man answered the phone, and we explained who we were looking for. He replied that there was no one in the operating room under that name. We were frantic. It was now 7:15 P.M. Where to turn next?

And then my sister-in-law remembered that she had been given a number to call for information. We found a pay phone and eventually reached the surgeon. He told us that the operation had ended at 3:00 P.M. and had been deemed a success.

Somewhat relieved, we were anxious to see her. Even that was not simple. After the operation, my mother-in-law had been moved to a different floor than the one she'd been on that morning. No one had told us that would happen.

As Unique As Snowflakes: Responding to Individuals

Every time I think of this, my blood pressure goes up. We'd just been sitting there like good little soldiers, waiting. I wonder when it would have dawned on someone to come and tell us that she was alive!

~

My teenage daughter had to have surgery on a Sunday morning. She had injured herself thirty-six hours earlier, and her knee was a mess. Waiting at home until the time for surgery arrived had been very stressful. My daughter had been in a lot of pain, and neither of us really knew how much damage had been done. Surgery would tell us that.

To some degree, I think we were both relieved when Sunday morning arrived. My daughter was exhausted from the pain, and I was exhausted from anxiety and from the surrogate pain of watching *her* pain.

I waited in a lounge on the same floor as the operating room. No one else was there. I didn't know what the surgeon would find when they opened up her knee. I had a book but couldn't concentrate enough to read. There was a jigsaw puzzle on the table, but I couldn't focus. I just shuffled through old magazines and checked my watch every ten minutes. An hour passed.

The next thing I remember is seeing a tall, slight woman, dressed in operating-room greens, coming through the door. She was smiling and exuded warmth as she held out her hand. "I'm the surgeon," she said, "and I'm pleased to report that the tissues around your daughter's knee were not torn—only seriously stretched. I was able to put everything back in place, and she's going to be right as rain in no time at all! You'll be able to see her in about an hour."

This surgeon put me completely at ease. Through her enthu- siasm, she communicated that she cared about my daughter. And because she was so happy with the results, I relaxed into a smile.

THE HEALING EFFECT
OF LISTENING

I'VE HAD THIS PERSISTENT SHORTNESS OF BREATH THAT HAPPENS MORE AND MORE FREQUENTLY. So I went to my family doctor, and she ordered a consult with a lung specialist. I went to him and had all sorts of tests. Word came back that, thank god, my lungs were fine. YAY! "But why can't I breathe?" I asked my family doctor.

Doctor: With a dull look and a shrug, "I'll send you to an ear-nose-throat specialist."

Me: "Is there anything else that may be causing this? It'll take months to get that appointment, and I'd like some relief soon."

Doctor: "Well, Dr. M. is a lung specialist, and he says there is nothing wrong with your lungs. He would know."

Me: "Yes, and I am glad of that. But I can't breathe. Any ideas?"

Doctor: Shrug . . . and more reading of Dr. M.'s notes.

Now, keep in mind, she had a patient sitting right in front of her—a patient who was telling her and showing her that she couldn't breathe well. And the doctor never looked. She just read the notes from the specialist. "Ah," I thought, "I guess the notes are more real than I am."

Today, I had another appointment with a different specialist—a cardio guy. This had been set up months earlier because of a family history of cardio stuff. The difference was night and day.

The Healing Effect of Listening

Me: "I know this isn't what you were consulted about, but I'm having this problem with breathing."

Cardiologist: Making eye contact and moving closer and listening, "Tell me about it." He took a great history and did a great exam.

Now remember—he wasn't originally consulted for lung stuff, but he decided that the patient in front of him was more important than the note from the family doctor. Imagine!

Cardiologist: "I can't see anything wrong with your lungs, so we have to cast the net wider. Have you ever had XYZ tests?"

Me: "No."

Cardiologist: "Well, how about we see what they show? I am sorry I can't find why you can't breathe."

We shook hands and said goodbye. I walked away and felt 100 percent better for having been respected and listened to.

Imagine—listening to the patient has a healing effect! Making eye contact! Paying heed! Recognizing that just because one option hasn't borne fruit, the patient is the first voice one should listen to. It all seems like it should be so damned simple.

TATTOO IT ON OUR HEARTS

IT WAS A HOLIDAY WEEKEND. My son and daughter-in-law were frantic when they called to say that their twenty-seven-month-old son was "screaming all the time." I urged them to take Benjamin to a doctor. They went to five different providers that weekend, all of whom said that they couldn't find anything. The parents kept saying that they'd never seen their son like this before, but the responses were all the same: "I'm the doctor, and there's nothing wrong with this child."

Finally, on Monday, my daughter-in-law Mary found a sixth doctor, who took an X-ray in his office. The X-ray identified an internal blockage (intussusception). He said that Benjamin needed to go to the hospital immediately.

At the time, I worked at a nearby hospital and so immediately went over to meet them. By the time the diagnosis came, my husband and son had arrived as well. The news was bad. Benjamin had cancer—a rhabdomyosarcoma of the bladder. This is a very aggressive tumor of soft tissue that was blocking his urethra and causing excruciatingly painful bladder spasms.

There were so many tests the first few days. Because Mary was pregnant, she couldn't be with Benjamin during the X-rays, and so Nathan, my son, went in with him. After the first MRI, Nathan came out sobbing. It turned out that the sight of Benjamin being anesthetized for this procedure was exactly like Nathan's freshly painful memories of putting his dog down three weeks earlier. He was not prepared for what he would see.

Benjamin was to have three weeks of chemotherapy to shrink the tumor and then have surgery to remove his bladder and cancer cells in all the margins. He would be in the hospital for about three weeks. There was a time when he had eleven tubes coming out of his body.

We did not want Benjamin to ever be alone. He was just a little guy, and there were lots of new, painful, and scary things happening to him. Because Mary was eight months pregnant, Nathan didn't think she should be alone, either at the hospital or at home. My son also felt that Mary should never drive home alone. And so we developed a plan: Nathan and Mary would stay at the hospital with Benjamin, and when they couldn't stay, my husband and I would stay.

And then we found out that the hospital had an "only one parent overnight" rule. We got the "one parent" lecture, and I asked the head nurse for the rationale for this policy. She told us it was because of fire regulations, but I was able to find out no such regulations existed. In the end, they allowed us to stay, but we never felt welcome.

One night, my husband and I stayed to give Mary and Nathan a break. I remember it vividly. Benjamin had an IV pump that beeped a few minutes before the IV bag needed to be changed. If you waited until the last minute, you would get a very persistent and loud beep. I wanted to avoid that because Benjamin had had a difficult day and I didn't want him to waken. I called the nurse and quietly explained my request. She came in, with a heavy sigh, and fixed the IV. On her way out, she slammed the door, waking Benjamin. I was able to settle him, but I was so angry, I was awake for hours. It was one of those little things I will never forget.

Did I do anything about it? No. We didn't want to rock the boat in any way, because these people were going to save our grandson's life, and we didn't want to make them angry.

Even though I held a senior position in nursing administration at another hospital, I always took my name tag off when I was visiting Benjamin. I wanted to be there as an ordinary grandmother, not as a nursing administrator. I felt intimidated in this new role on the receiving end of care. I found myself trying to be sure not to do anything wrong.

But the problem was we didn't really know the rules. For example, Mary and Nathan, not wanting to leave the unit, usually ate in the hallway, outside Benjamin's room, at an unused table. Apparently, eating in the hallway broke some rule, but no one told us about it or told us what our alternative was. All we got were cold stares.

Family members of other patients were the ones who told us the most. They told us how things worked, who to avoid, what the rules were, and more. For example, in the intensive care unit family waiting area, there was a sign that said "Only two visitors at a time, and visiting only twenty minutes per hour." But other parents told us, "Oh, you don't need to worry about that. They don't really follow that. Just stay out of their way." Even though I'd been a nurse for years, I had never understood that family members know as much as they do.

I also learned that, typically, doctors and nurses have no idea what effect a disease like this has on a family at home. Mary and Nathan had to learn to manage complex procedures and equipment such as IVs and total parenteal nutrition (TPN) tubes. And then there was the sheer volume of medical supplies, equipment, and IV pumps that were needed on site for Benjamin's care. Even as a health care professional with years of experience, I was overwhelmed.

Layered on top of worrying about and caring for Benjamin, Nathan and Mary were burdened by financial pressures. Prior to Benjamin's getting sick, they both had two jobs to make ends meet. Just to manage the care regime, they had to give up their evening jobs and therefore lost income. They also had additional expenses for all the things they needed for home care. They finally moved in with us to have some hands-on help and general support.

The silver lining in this whole experience was how much I learned as a health care professional. I learned how to relate to families in ways that are genuinely helpful. I learned that the best professionals are those who are open to sharing what they know *and* what they don't. I learned about asking patients what was important to them rather than telling them what was important to me. And I learned that when people and families come to us, we cannot separate their physical bodies from their emotional and social worlds.

More than anything else, I learned that all of us who work in health care should recall the platinum rule, which says, "Do unto others as they want you to do." We should tattoo it on our hearts.

AN ENORMOUS BURDEN IS LIFTED

I CANNOT ADEQUATELY DESCRIBE HOW I FELT. I had just said goodbye to my daughter, Mary. She was taking the ferry to go to Vancouver and, from there, to catch the plane back to Toronto. I did not know if I would ever see her again.

By this point, Mary was terribly thin again and was becoming weaker every day. She had turned down an opportunity to enter the eating disorders program at Toronto General Hospital a couple of months earlier but now had decided to give it and herself a chance. I ached to go with her, but we both knew she had to do this on her own. This time it had to be for herself.

Our roller-coaster journey with anorexia was now in its second year. The ride started slowly at first and then gathered speed. Our family of four quickly realized that we were caught by a force over which we had no control. We all desperately tried to grasp for something to hold on to and things to blame. We searched for patterns, causes, cures, and hints of hope.

When Mary was first admitted to the pediatric hospital's program for children with eating disorders, we all hoped this would help. We were terribly worried, but also, in a sense, relieved. We had admitted that this problem was bigger than anything any of us, alone or together, could manage. One of the components of the program, like most eating-disorder programs, was family counseling.

Contrary to their intended effect, I can't state strongly enough how damaging these family counseling sessions were. Not only were they of no help to Mary, but the message communicated to the rest of us—me and her father and brother—was that we were all to blame, "because these kinds of problems do not occur in a vacuum." This had the effect of digging the tunnel of my deepest fear—that something about my parenting had caused this horrible situation. My husband chose to deflect blame away from himself. He became more insistent and emboldened in his belief that Mary's problems were my fault, because I had not made Mary eat breakfast every morning when she was eleven. And my son, angered that some stranger had implicated him as part of his beloved sister's problem, withdrew into himself, like a turtle protecting its soft inner core.

Mary was ultimately released from the hospital. She had gained enough weight but clearly had not gained the kind of understanding or peace of mind that would allow her to love herself enough to want to live. The roller-coaster ride continued. Mary had good days and bad days, my marriage fell apart, and my son managed to continue to achieve at school but became listless. My days were cloaked in a mantle of guilt, the weight of which left me with a feeling of powerlessness in terms of helping Mary or reaching out to my son.

But I did read, and I talked to people. I learned enough about eating disorders to understand, at least intellectually, that watching Mary like a hawk and trying to have just the right kinds of food in the house would not really make any difference. I learned that some anorexics have to get to their lowest point possible before they can begin their road back. I learned that I had to let go of the situation, that even if I had been a cause, I could not be a cure.

For example, Mary said that she needed some time alone and wanted to visit a favorite older friend on Vancouver Island. I had to say yes. If I'd created this situation because of being overprotective, I now had to bend the other way. When I joined her several days later, I could see that Mary was getting worse. This was when she said she was ready to go into the program in Toronto.

And that was the day that I gently hugged her fragile body, told her I loved her, and waved goodbye as she headed for the ferry. She called me a couple of days later from Toronto saying she could get into the program in ten days, but she didn't know if she could last that long. She asked me to join her.

By the time Mary was admitted to the hospital, she was in terrible shape. Four days later, as I was helping support her in the bathroom, she collapsed in my arms. Her heart was failing her. She looked at me with terrified eyes and said, "Mom, please tell me stories." For the next three hours, I spoke without stopping.

I told her the stories of "Little Red Riding Hood" and "Three Billy Goats Gruff," two tales I had told her many times when she was little. But mostly, I told her family stories—going back to my grandparents, and how they ended up in Canada, and all the happenings in between, and how her dad and I got together, and what it was like the day she was born, and all sorts of remembrances of her when she was tiny.

As Mary fought for her life, I basically reconstructed her through narrative. I created a tapestry of her life by weaving colorful and comforting strands of stories. It was intense, and she held my hand in a vice grip while connected to tubes and monitors of all kinds. Eventually, after almost three hours, Mary's breathing changed. I raised my eyes in panic, silently asking the nurse, who had been present throughout, what was happening. She responded gently, "It's okay. She's sleeping now." And then I had the luxury of weeping.

A pivotal event for Mary had taken place. She had, in that moment of physiological crisis, chosen to live. She had hit bottom and had begun to return from her own place of darkness. It wasn't going to be an easy path, but she had clearly set her compass, her own true north. It was shortly after this that I managed to turn a corner myself, and I will never forget the moment it occurred.

Mary and I met with her new psychiatrist some days after her medical crisis had stabilized. Within the first five minutes with this doctor, forever to be a saint in my eyes, he made it clear that with eating disorders there was to be no blame; no one was responsible for this; guilt should not be part of anyone's vocabulary. The sensations I felt were profound, like the first sip of water must feel to one who has been lost in a desert for days on end, like the first flapping of a butterfly's wing when it has just emerged from a tightly wrapped cocoon, like the first glimmer of light a miner sees when rescued from a mine shaft of darkness.

This whole journey has been full of pain, worry, confusion, and fear. It did not need to have guilt added to the existing complexity of emotions. I try my best to be positive and to be thankful for the opportunities that have been provided for all of us to know ourselves better and to relate to each other with greater sensitivity and compassion. But it has been a long, bleak journey made more difficult by a professional who failed to understand that when a child is seriously ill, families are vulnerable and need support, not attacks, to triumph over adversity that tests everyone to the core.

WHERE'S THE HEADACHE?

WHEN I WAS ALONE AT OUR COTTAGE, I THOUGHT I WAS HAVING A HEART ATTACK. I called 911. The paramedics determined that I was okay but told me to follow up with my family doctor.

I saw my family doctor two weeks later. I told him what had happened and also mentioned that I'd been having severe headaches. He took my blood pressure, told me it was very high, and said, "Go to the hospital right away."

I went to the emergency room. By the time I got there, my blood pressure had decreased a bit and so I wasn't considered critical. I was told to wait.

I waited because my doctor had told me to go to the hospital. I'm fifty, I'm overweight, and I'm a smoker. I know all that puts me at risk for trouble. I was scared.

I waited eleven hours and was eventually put in a little cubicle lined with curtains. And then I heard the doctor say, "Where's the headache?" I had been reduced to a symptom. I was no longer a person with a name.

When the doctor came in to see me, he let me know that he was annoyed with my doctor for sending me to the hospital. He said it had been a frivolous waste of resources. He made me feel like I was a hypochondriac, just wanting attention.

I wish he had called my doctor instead of yelling at me. I was just doing what I'd been told.

I'M THE FULL-TIME TENANT
OF THIS BODY

SEPTEMBER 27, 2004. Simple enough. I was leaving work and heading to the parking lot to get my car. I was crossing a busy street. Halfway across, the light changed and I started running. And that's when I was hit. I'm told I flew ten to fifteen feet before I landed.

The ambulance took me to the emergency department. I was holding my arm and saying my leg hurt too. They said that the X-rays showed a broken wrist and a crack in my leg. They thought the wrist might need surgery, but I was told that if I didn't put too much weight on my leg, it would probably heal. I was sent home with one crutch and an appointment to see an orthopedic surgeon two days later.

It was ultimately determined that I needed surgery on both my wrist and my knee. The crack in my leg was, in fact, right into the knee joint—a radial spiral fracture and a plateau fracture. Surgery was scheduled.

The operation took place in the afternoon. I woke up in the evening. I called the nurse because I was in a lot of pain and said, "My leg feels swollen." She said, "Of course, you've just had surgery." My leg kept getting more and more painful. I kept calling the nurses, and they kept saying, "You've just had an operation—this is normal." Around midnight, the nurses even convinced my wife to go home to get some sleep, saying, "The worst is over."

But by 2 A.M., my foot was enormous and my leg felt like it was exploding, being crushed from the inside out. Now I had three nurses in my room looking very concerned. One of them was on a cell phone calling a doctor. They couldn't find a pulse in my foot.

It turned out that one of the screws that had been put into my knee had nicked an artery at the back of the knee and had been bleeding into my leg for hours. A surgical team was assembled. The pain was excruciating.

By 7 A.M., I was being rolled into the operating room again, this time to replace the screws, to repair the artery, and to make an incredibly long incision down my shin to relieve the pressure. Fortunately, someone made a judgment call not to send me for a preoperative angiogram. The surgeon later reflected, "If the bleeding had gone on any longer, we'd have lost your foot."

I was in the intensive care unit (ICU) for three days. I was still in a lot of pain. My wife Christy slept in the ICU. She would tell me every time six minutes passed so that I could push the button for pain medication. I felt like she was my lifeline. I can still remember the terrible moment when, just after Christy had gone to the hospital cafeteria to get some dinner, my nurse came to tell me that she was leaving to do a shift change. I felt totally abandoned and had a complete panic attack. I wouldn't have made it without my wife.

I remember the vascular surgeon visiting me and my alien leg every day. He had a grave, concerned look on his face. I tried to lighten him up. I wondered why this guy was so serious. It took a while to dawn on me that the surgeon was serious because he didn't know if I'd still lose my foot.

But as the vascular situation improved and people stopped worrying about any need to amputate, I began to experience a different kind of pain. As a result of the extraordinary swelling from the internal bleeding, it seems that the nerves in my leg had been crushed. What I was starting to feel was the knife-piercing sensations of nerve pain.

I'm the Full-Time Tenant of This Body

For two weeks this pain escalated to the point that the nerve medications could not be increased any further. Even with maximum medication, a person's breath on my foot was more than I could bear. Finally the pain peaked and began to subside. Apparently, nerves—if they're going to regenerate—regrow at the rate of one millimeter a day. Given the distance between my knee and my foot, it will take two years to fully recover from this damage. I have another year to go.

After four weeks, I had more surgery to close the wounds and apply a skin graft. Finally, I was able to go home, with a walker fitted with an armrest (because of my broken wrist).

There are a few things that stand out from my hospital stay:

♦ I remember calling the nurses one night with my call button. I had to call three times before anyone answered. They'd turned me off. You know, you can say you're busy, but don't turn me off. I've worked in customer service for too long to find this acceptable.

♦ Two nurses were great. One was friendly and would just stop in and take a bit of time to talk. She'd offer to get my wife juice. Another one, a career nurse from Oklahoma, also took time to talk and share a bit of herself. She'd also listen to what I had to say. Acknowledging me (and my wife) made the difference between a good nurse and a mediocre one.

♦ It was gratifying when people gave me credit for knowing things. After all, I am the full-time tenant of my body. I'm here all the time, not just for a ten-hour shift. I'm a relatively smart guy, and I was paying attention to what was happening to me. I was learning a lot. I remember knowing enough to stop a nurse once from drawing blood in an inappropriate position.

♦ A positive attitude is so important. It's not always easy, and the days when I couldn't bring my mind up from the depths of despair were the hardest. Sometimes you need help to be positive because you're so exhausted.

♦ Oddly enough, I was fond of my orthopedic surgeon. It's very challenging to juxtapose this with all that I've been through and what I still live with every day, but he has a nice, easygoing manner. He'd always tell me everything that he was doing. After things went wrong, he was very gracious and made sure I got the best care I could get in terms of vascular surgery, plastic surgery, infectious disease issues, and pain management. He was kind. He was always willing to listen to my concerns and put forth some effort to get what I needed.

While I was recuperating at home, I went to the burn clinic as an outpatient for graft therapy. On one of these visits, a nurse said, "I think this is looking a little red and warm." And so off I went to see the plastic surgeon, who poked at the skin graft. It exploded! So back I went to surgery to have my wound flushed and cleaned.

By the beginning of December, I was beginning to put a bit of weight on my leg. On Christmas day, I threw down my crutches and joked, "It's a Christmas miracle." You know, if you don't laugh, you have to cry. The whole thing was so overwhelming and serious—I couldn't focus on that—making light of the situation helped me cope.

How am I now? My wrist is okay and I walk with a tiny limp. My leg is strong enough so that I can run on a soft surface. I still have some weird nerve sensations. Will I have problems resulting from this in ten or twenty years? I don't know.

I'm the Full-Time Tenant of This Body

I know people tell me things like, "You're walking so much earlier than we thought," but I think it's not soon enough. Or they say, "You're making such good progress," but I think I shouldn't have to be going through this at all.

And what will I tell my new little son about all this when he grows up? I'll tell him to look both ways before he crosses the street! I'll tell him to be careful out there! And maybe I'll tell him that my amazing scars are from a shark attack or a snowboarding accident when I was in the Alps!

This young man chose not to sue for medical malpractice. He explained that he was already dealing with other legal issues regarding insurance and workers compensation claims stemming from the accident. Additionally, as he says, "While a mistake had been made, proving that it was malpractice would have been expensive, time consuming, and possibly futile. Also, the surgeon is a nice guy and I didn't feel compelled to attack him."

THE VALUE OF ASKING QUESTIONS

In December 2002, my Christmas present to my eighty-year-old mother was an ambulance transport to move her to Massachusetts from a hospital in New York. It was a dramatic event, but I felt it was necessary to save her life. My parents had lived in New York their entire lives, and so this step was not taken lightly.

It's important to explain that my mom had a passion for learning. She was a bright, intelligent, analytical woman. She was a homemaker and community activist, offering advice and help to everyone. She had asked for a computer for her eightieth birthday. She used this tool to keep herself intellectually sharp and connected to her community.

That December, my mother had to go to the hospital for a surgical procedure. I was living in Massachusetts at the time but still managed to visit her every two or three days. The hospital staff would express their frustrations about my mother. They said that she had many questions about the side effects of the medications she was receiving and was asking about alternative therapies.

In my experience with older patients, health care providers are often not as respectful of a patient's and family's ability to ask questions. I even felt that my own engagement as a family-based advocate was not well received. I encouraged the staff to take my mother's concerns seriously, telling them that she was very observant and inquisitive by nature. In addition, I felt it was her right to expect respectful answers to her questions regarding her own treatment.

I am a physician myself, so I was in a difficult situation. On the one hand, as a son, I was experiencing the emotional ramifications of seeing my mother in distress. On the other hand, as a professional, I kept seeing the real potential for errors in medical judgment. In addition to my mother's questions, I would also ask questions, usually in response to an overt or impending mistake. For example, one night I saw that an error was about to occur with managing her fluid intake. Rather than challenging the physician directly, I asked questions and made a suggestion for a different approach. He commented that I knew "quite a bit about adult medicine for a pediatrician!"

On Christmas Eve, I noticed that my mother was extremely sedated. I asked what had happened. A nurse came up to me and whispered, "Please don't tell anyone I told you this because I could get into trouble. A consulting doctor has put your mother on Haldol." I couldn't believe what I was hearing. No one in the family was notified about this recommendation. My mother was too ill to give her consent. I knew that Haldol was one of the most powerful antipsychotic drugs, and that it was inappropriate to use in a postsurgical, eighty-year-old woman whose agitation was caused solely by poorly controlled pain. That's when I booked the ambulance transport to bring her to our community in Massachusetts.

Once that crisis was behind us, and my mom and dad were settled into living in our home, I began to look for a primary care provider for my parents. I wanted to find someone who embraced the same values that I try to bring to my own pediatric medical practice—someone who believed in the family's right and privilege to contribute to their own care and care planning, and someone who viewed the family as a full partner in a two-way relationship.

It wasn't as easy as I would have liked it to be. We found many physicians who had no idea what it means to be family-centered and had no desire to learn. It took about a year, but we finally put together what we thought was a good team for my mother's health care. As it turned out, our expectations for my mother's primary care provider were not fulfilled.

Mom was diagnosed with ovarian cancer. As was her way, she had a lot of questions about the proposed treatments, their side effects, and whether there were any alternatives. The day before she was to start chemotherapy, she received a registered letter from her primary care doctor.

This was a registered letter—not a phone call. The letter said that the primary care physician was releasing my mother from his practice because she had been asking too many questions. He said, "The only people who stay in my care are those who do exactly what I tell them." He allowed no opportunity to question or attempt to reach a collaborative strategy. In fact, he felt threatened by the concept of a family-professional partnership.

As difficult as this challenge was to our family, imposed the day before a grueling course of chemotherapy was to begin, it motivated us to develop proactive strategies to deal with the limitations of a health care system that was not particularly sensitive to the intellectual or emotional needs of its consumers.

During my mother's chemotherapy, we were able to engage a new primary care provider. This physician embraced the concept of partnership. She celebrated my mother's cognitive abilities and affirmed her right to ask questions. This ultimately led to a collaboration invigorated by mutual respect. It led to the creation of a care plan that honored my mother's choices, dignity, and quality of life. It brought out family strengths that enabled us to endure very challenging times, including accepting a terminal diagnosis. Clearly, this physician understood that collaboratively planned treatment with dignity is more valuable than an autocratic approach to "cure." Cultivating a family's strengths is an ultimate goal of any effective family-professional partnership. We were blessed to have found a doctor who endorsed this philosophy.

Dr. Richard Antonelli is Chief of the Division of Primary Care and Director of the Department of General Pediatrics at the Connecticut Children's Medical Center at the University of Connecticut School of Medicine. He is committed to a process of care delivery called Medical Home. It has been endorsed by the American Academy of Pediatrics, the National Association of Pediatric Nurse Practitioners, and the American Academy of Family Physicians and strives to ensure that every child and youth, especially those with special health needs, receive health care that is family-centered, comprehensive, compassionate, continuous, coordinated, accessible, and culturally competent. In this model, the family is the acknowledged expert in the child's care.

Dr. Antonelli says, "This approach to care is what I try to put in place for my patients. It should be the norm in adult medicine as well." When asked how he came to this view as a doctor, he replied, "Respecting families as partners is fundamentally important. It starts in your heart. I can honestly say that families have been some of my most influential teachers in the twenty-five years that I have been in medicine." He goes on to say, "The health care system must exist to serve the needs of families, not the reverse. Families must be thought of as full partners in advising on matters of quality, compassion, and cultural effectiveness."

Dr. Antonelli's mother, Evelyn, died on September 9, 2005, three days following this interview. Dr. Antonelli shared with his mother that her story would be told. Mrs. Antonelli was able to appreciate the value of having her story used to inspire other families to expect nothing less than full partnership with their health care providers.

Being Together:
The Power of Family

"I am sure I only survived because of my doctor's
great care and my parents' great love."
—Pamela Stein

"Life loves to be taken by the lapel and told:
'I'm with you kid. Let's go.'"
—Maya Angelou

"One thing you realize when you're sick
is that you aren't the only person who needs support—
sometimes you have to be the one who supports others."
—Lance Armstrong

∼

When we're ill or injured, don't we all want our family
and friends around us? It's family and friends who know
us, who can speak for us if we have lost our voices,
who know what calms us, who know what we can do,
who will be there to help us in the long run.
And stories from patients and families can help
health care providers see where seeds of hope
or despair are planted.

Just as patients and families need support, so do health
care professionals. Their close working relationships
often create a sense of "family" at work.
When these "families" are threatened, then staff
need as much support as patients and families.

I WANT MY CHILDREN WITH ME
SMILES TELL THE STORY
OLIVIA'S STORY
IT WAS AS HARD AS IT GETS

I WANT MY CHILDREN WITH ME

*This Canadian mother was travelling with her four children
on a ski vacation in the United States. Black ice led
to a dreadful accident in which two of her children were killed
instantly and one of the other two, her daughter, suffered a
deep laceration on her face, along with a broken arm
and a broken bone in her foot. The mother, with a broken
sternum and humerus, was in excruciating pain.
Somehow, in the chaos of the moment and in spite of the
overwhelming nature of the tragedy and of her own pain,
the mother remembers a great deal of the first
minutes, hours, and days.*

IT WAS A SUNNY, WINTER DAY—NOT THE KIND OF DAY YOU WOULD EXPECT AN ACCIDENT. But black ice knows no rules, and, as if controlled by an unseeing hand moving in slow motion, our car and a plow truck crashed into each other. Two cars, eight people; two dead, two injured, four emotionally traumatized.

Like a mother lioness, I fought to control what I could, fighting through the physical pain of a twice-broken arm and a smashed sternum and the emotional agony of knowing, instantly, that two of my four children lay dead in the surrounding bushes.

I held my youngest daughter, Chrissie, with my good arm and tried to assess her injuries. At the same time, I tried to calm my oldest son. Scott, a new, young driver, had been driving at the time of the accident and was terribly shaken and upset. He knew that Chrissie and I were injured and in pain and had already discovered that his two other siblings were in the surrounding brush, having been thrown from the car, dying on impact.

As my son gave voice to his own agony and guilt by saying, "Mom, I want to kill myself," I firmly replied, "Scott, I've just lost Nancy and Nate; I can't lose you, too." Little did I know I would be echoing this theme within the hour.

When the state troopers arrived, I asked them to speak to my son. I remember that the state troopers were so kind to take my distraught son aside to assure him that the accident had not been his fault, that it truly had been an accident. They made the same statement to the local media, all of which was ultimately a huge comfort to Scott.

At the scene of the accident, I made it very clear to the ambulance drivers that Chrissie and I should be taken to the same hospital. When I arrived at the hospital, however, Chrissie was not there. The emergency room staff were very accommodating, and wheeled my stretcher to phones so that I could talk to my daughter's doctor at another hospital.

The doctor at the other hospital told me he wanted to operate on Chrissie right away, but I countered, saying that I wanted my daughter brought to the hospital where I was. The doctor retorted, "Well, you obviously don't understand. If your daughter is moved, I can't take any responsibility for what happens to her."

Speaking tersely, through teeth clenched from both pain and anger, I said, "In fact I do understand, doctor. I understand that I've just lost two of my children, and I want my others with me, here, now." And then I asked, "Doctor, are you telling me it's a matter of life and death as to whether my daughter can be moved?"

"No, just that I won't take any responsibility for anything happening to her if she is moved."

"That's fine, doctor—I'll take full responsibility!"

One of the paramedics, having overheard my side of the conversation, reassured me by saying, "Don't you worry ma'am! I'll go get her."

Meanwhile, the staff at my hospital were sensitive and caring enough to get Scott a stretcher so that he could lie down beside my stretcher and talk with me, eye to eye, quietly, privately. He asked, "Mum, are you going to be okay?" I answered, "If you mean am I going to die, then no, I'm not going to die. I'm badly injured, but I'm going to be okay."

I was so touched by the empathetic responses of the staff at this small city hospital. I knew that the nurses were upset because I could see their tears. I knew that the ambulance driver understood my anguish about being separated from my daughter, as he had so quickly volunteered to pick her up from the other hospital. And I could see that the young doctor on call was gently crying, and I knew he understood, because he had children the same ages as mine. I remember him saying, his eyes glistening, "I hate to ask you this, but could you please try not to cry. We're concerned your lung might collapse."

The hospital, with my permission, allowed the husband and wife who had been in the other vehicle—a plow truck—to see me while I was still in emergency. The woman was a nurse; she and her husband had children of their own. They were both overcome with the tragedy of the situation. Aware of their grief and sense of guilt, I tried to emotionally reach out to them and tell them that it hadn't been their fault. I think being able to see them was an important part of my own healing.

Eventually, Chrissie was brought to the hospital where Scott and I had been waiting for her. Surgery was scheduled right away for Chrissie, and the plastic surgeon explained everything to me. I was able to stay with her until she went to the operating room and was in a room across the hall when she came back from the operation.

While Chrissie was in surgery, I began to try to find out where Nancy and Nate were. Sadly, there was an atmosphere of secrecy, as apparently no one had the right to convey the truth. I pleaded with the nurses, saying, "I know they're dead. I just want to hold them one more time." It was only when the coroner arrived that I learned my children's bodies had been taken to the morgue, and I would not be able to see them. This was not the answer I wanted, but at least I had an answer.

Scott and I were taken upstairs to a big room with lots of bright windows. A phone was handy. No one ever raised the subject of money, of how much all this was going to cost, of whether I could pay.

A social worker called a priest and helped make all the arrangements for the air ambulance to take Chrissie and me home to Canada. She also helped find other people for me to talk with. Clearly, it was acknowledged that I wanted to try to still be in control, to still make all the decisions on my own. For example, I talked with the coroner about whether Nancy and Nate should be embalmed immediately in order to have a choice in terms of whether the family would want to have open caskets.

After Chrissie's surgery, she and I were able to spend the night together in the same room. The nurses cleverly put the two beds together in such a way that her good hand could reach out to hold my foot all through the night.

Within forty-eight hours, arrangements had been made to get everyone home to Canada. I recall that the air ambulance men were very kind and sensitive. They seemed to know how much every movement sent waves of intense pain through my body and tried to be as careful as possible. They also brought Chrissie a teddy bear to have and to hug. However, there were some things they couldn't do.

For example, I had asked for enough pain medication to get me through the whole trip by air, including the time I would have to wait on the ground to clear customs and immigration in Canada. As it turned out, however, I was only given enough medication for the duration of the flight itself, and no one on the air ambulance had the authority to administer morphine. Tragically, literally adding insult to injury, my pain was allowed to get out of control unnecessarily.

At home, two hospitals had been alerted that a local woman and her daughter were being flown in from the United States. In spite of the forewarning, a communication breakdown occurred when I arrived at my hospital. Even though the hospital had actually assigned an inpatient private room for me, I was still taken to a cubicle in emergency and told to wait. To me, it seemed as if no one knew what was going on. After what seemed forever, someone came in and started asking a series of questions, such as, "What is your full name?" and "What is your phone number?" Writhing in pain, I snapped, yelling, "I'm not supposed to be here. Call someone!"

Unlike the hospital, the local media knew exactly what they were waiting for, and they behaved like hungry piranhas. Scott and his father had to be taken through the airport via hidden entrances and exits to avoid the media mob. Relentlessly, the media finally tracked Scott down, calling him at home and hounding him with questions about what caused the accident and how he felt about it all. Privacy was not something the media respected. All they wanted was a story.

Eventually the media went away, this mother's bones knitted together, her daughter's surgery to repair facial lacerations healed, and her son resumed driving. But emotional pain does not go away. Memories remain vivid, and included in those are the people who tried to soothe a family literally torn apart by a dreadful accident and the people whose actions poured unwanted salt into wrenching wounds.

SMILES TELL THE STORY

MY SOUL WAS MOVED TODAY. We have a husband and wife as patients in our intensive care unit who were in a terrible motor vehicle collision that killed a member of their family. They were both critically injured themselves, and both are on ventilators.

While I was making rounds this morning, I noted the incredible silence in the unit. I also noted that the nurses and respiratory therapist were gathered around a patient's bed.

As I drew closer, I saw that the staff had taken the husband off of his ventilator (bagging him instead) and pushed his bed next to his wife's bed so that they could touch each other for the first time since they came here ten days ago. Although they couldn't turn to look at each other, their smiles told their story of gratitude and love.

I am so proud to be part of a place that values kindness as an integral component of care.

OLIVIA'S STORY

*A mother shares her concerns about her daughter's hospital stay
through a letter to the hospital's administration.*

DEAR SIR,

When Olivia was born she was placed in my arms, and I was
told, "You have a seven-pound, healthy baby girl." Five weeks
later, I was trying to convince the doctor that there was something terribly wrong.

We learned that Olivia had a one-pound tumor in her
abdomen that had to be removed. I had not even had a chance
to be a good mother to her when I had to turn her over to
strangers.

The surgery lasted about six hours, after which she was in the
recovery room for several hours more. We did not get to see her
in the recovery room. She was eventually transferred to the pediatric intensive care unit (PICU). We were permitted to see her at
5:00 P.M., the first time in ten hours.

At 5:00 the next morning, we called the unit to see how she
was. We repeatedly got a busy signal, so we just drove to the hospital. When we arrived, we were told that the doctors were still
doing rounds, and, therefore, we could not visit Olivia.

After rounds were over, I called the unit again to ask permission to visit and was told to wait "just a little longer." I waited and
then called again and was told to wait another twenty minutes. I
kept calling every twenty minutes, and each time I was put off.
At one point, I was told they were doing some surgery and I
would have to wait. They didn't know how long it would be.

Olivia's Story

I had been anxious up to that point, but then I got really frightened. I asked what the problem was, and all I was told was that they were working on my baby and I should call back later. It was now 2:00 P.M., and I hadn't seen my baby for twenty hours! Not only was I frantic—I was also getting very angry. Finally, I called again and simply said I was coming in.

When I got inside the PICU, I found that the place where Olivia's crib had been was empty. I panicked! Then I saw her crib being rolled out the opposite end of the unit, and I ran to it. The nurses were very lighthearted, saying, "We're taking her to the floor. Isn't that great?" I saw that someone had glued a pink bow to the top of my baby's head, and I just lost it!

It's hard to describe what went through my mind at the time. The nurses had no time for me to come in to visit my baby because they were too busy with other critical patients, but they had time to play with her hair and glue a bow to her head. I wanted to scream, "I'm her mother! I want to be the one to play with her, to put her first bow in her hair. Who do you think you are, taking over my child as though I'm unimportant and in the way?"

I was furious, and the nurses couldn't understand why I was so angry. I wondered if any of them had children of their own. I wondered if any of them knew what it feels like to have your baby pulled from your arms and completely controlled by strangers who sat at the end of a phone line saying, "Just wait a little longer."

The last time I had seen Olivia, she had tubes everywhere and was connected to a bank of machines, including a ventilator. When did all this equipment come off? Why wasn't I told that she was improving? I had made it very clear that I wanted to know what was being done to my child. I had called repeatedly. The nurses and doctors had every opportunity to tell me what was happening to my baby, even if they wouldn't let me in. Who do they think they are that they can completely ignore the rights and concerns of parents? Was there any need to continually prove to us they were in control, and we were not?

Later, Olivia was readmitted to the PICU, and we went through the same calling routine again. It seems senseless to me that only one nurse can decide if I can see my child, and, if so, when and for how long. No explanations, no logical reasoning—just "no!"

If there had been more information given to me that had made sense, I could have waited better. I know that nurses and doctors have to do their job, but part of their job is me. Babies don't come to hospitals alone. They have parents. I was only allowed to visit when I became irate, and so every time I went into the unit, I was irate. What way is that to establish rapport with a family?

I look forward to hearing from you.

Sincerely,
A Concerned Mother

In this hospital's case, the hospital administrator was stunned when she received this letter. In a very real sense, she was grateful that this mother took the time to write, because she learned that practices on the floors were not as she thought they were. She used this mother's letter to improve care and change the way that staff worked with families. A clear commitment was made to family-centered care and to the education of all staff so that the situations described in the letter would never happen again to another family.

IT WAS AS HARD AS IT GETS:
The Impact of a Global Crisis on Family-Centered Care

SARS. SEVERE ACUTE RESPIRATORY SYNDROME. Even today, the term provokes a profound response from those who were closest to the outbreak.

SARS is a severe type of pneumonia that is rapidly progressive and sometimes fatal. SARS is highly communicable and is spread by direct and droplet contact.

In the early months of 2003, SARS appeared as a new infectious disease. It originated in China and became a disease of global proportion in a relatively short period of time. International travel made it easy for the disease to move from country to country. Cases were reported in 29 countries, and there were 774 deaths worldwide.

On March 7, 2003, Toronto, Canada, had its first identified hospital case of SARS. By March 26, a provincial emergency was declared. On April 23, the World Health Organization issued a travel advisory (in effect for only 6 days). The provincial state of emergency continued until May 18. And then a second outbreak of SARS occurred on May 22 and the crisis didn't wane until August 2003.

During the acute phase of the outbreak, the Ontario Ministry of Health imposed strict guidelines with a single focus of wanting to protect patients, families, and staff. Many decisions, designed to provide safety for the greatest number of people, resulted in a terrible push-pull between the losses of some individual rights and the larger context of protecting the public good.

The severity of the guidelines varied from hospital to hospital, depending on the number of staff who had become sick with SARS. Hospitals were rated according to a numerical scale. In hospitals where no staff had become sick with SARS, the rating was low and the guidelines were less restrictive than in hospitals where staff had become sick.

For example, in a hospital where no staff were sick with SARS, non-SARS patients could have one visitor. By comparison, non-SARS patients in hospitals where staff were sick with SARS were not allowed any visitors at all. Patients with SARS were not allowed any visitors, no matter what the hospital's rating. The different ratings and corresponding rules created confusion for the public.

Many hospital and health care professionals in Ontario hospitals were passionately committed to collaborating with and involving patients and families in care. They had worked long and hard to bring about positive changes in institutional and staff attitudes and practices and then suddenly found these gains compromised, overwhelmed, and paralyzed by forces beyond their control. While controlling the outbreak and protecting people from harm were the objectives, there were significant consequences.

Overnight, hospitals and care practices went from being family-centered to system-centered. Overnight, hospitals went into what felt like a lockdown mentality: Entry points were limited, all patients and staff were screened for symptoms, and security personnel made sure no one got past the front door. Overnight, many families were told they could not be with their loved ones. Overnight, the support, information, and additional care families typically provided was no longer easily available to staff, overruled by infection-control priorities. Overnight, all volunteers and several categories of staff, including psychologists and chaplains, were declared non-essential and were prevented from coming to work. Overnight, health care professionals became bigger, taller, wider, and more removed from their patients because of protective clothing. Overnight, people became afraid.

It Was As Hard As It Gets

In the world of pediatric medicine, it is common for parents to stay with a hospitalized child. During the SARS outbreak, however, if a child had been exposed to SARS, the child would typically be whisked away in an ambulance and that child's parents were not allowed to enter the hospital. If a child was hospitalized for a non-SARS reason but a parent had been exposed to SARS, the parents were denied access to the hospital. Nurses reported that they couldn't bear hearing children, from small babies to teenagers, crying because they wanted their mothers and fathers.

Staff would do their best to make up for parents' absence and facilitate some sort of communication between child and family. Staff would take pictures and send them home; they would ask for pictures of family members to be sent in. Cards would be mailed and e-mails would be sent. Phones became critically important to families trying to stay in touch and provide support for each other. Some calls would last for hours, with parents at home providing comfort for children undergoing procedures, and children being reassured that their family members at home or in other hospitals were still healthy and alive.

Hospital-wide precautions required children to be confined to their rooms. All playrooms were closed. In such conditions of isolation and boredom, children often became depressed and anxious. Child life specialists did their best to find ways for children to play and overcome this new profound sense of being cooped up.

Special toss- and target-style games were created; the closed-circuit television system was used for group games like Bingo; and one child life specialist even arranged for children to sit at the entrances to their rooms where they could at least see and interact with others and play verbal trivia games. Additionally, some of the volunteers no longer allowed access to the hospital made craft kits off-site to be delivered to isolated children to work on in their rooms.

Various stories from adult hospitals convey some of the tragic side effects of this outbreak. For example, a female patient in intensive care was unable to talk and was going blind. Her husband had been with her nonstop. Overnight, he was told he would no longer be allowed to visit his wife. Desperate to communicate, he e-mailed his wife daily love letters which the staff would read to her and then laugh and cry together.

In one excruciating situation, all members of a single family had been exposed to and become sick with SARS. Tragically, they were all in different hospitals, sick themselves and worried about the others. Staff from these different hospitals did their best to be in touch with each other and to convey information and messages of hugs and comfort.

The mother of an eighteen-year-old boy who had been in a car accident begged to be able to stay with her son. He had been a bright, intelligent young man and had suffered a terrible head injury. He was just starting to communicate again. The mother was completely prepared to waive her rights to safety to be with her son and help him recover, but she was told she had no rights to waive. The system was larger than her love.

A calm, reasonable, rational, dignified immigrant woman, already struggling to adjust to a different culture and language, lost all composure when she was told and finally understood that she could not visit her sister. She was forcibly restrained by security staff until she could bottle up and contain her personal agony.

Hospital staff had to wear special clothing, including face shields and masks Smiles designed to try to brighten a dark day were hidden from view. Patients could not even recognize a nurse they knew until that person spoke. Staff talked about how difficult it was to not be able to provide the comfort of touch to patients because there was always a protective layer of clothing in the way. Many reported feelings of guilt; because the striker suits were so hot, staff desperately wanted to just get out of their patients' rooms to be able to breathe again. Others described they felt "fog, fatigue, and exhaustion" from wearing masks for twelve hours.

Compassionate staff were caught in this web of complexity. They tried their best to keep patient and family lines of communication open and to show kindness in the midst of delivering care. And yet all the while they were terribly aware that when patients are not surrounded by the support of family, their recovery is diminished.

Staff also talked about how hard it was to do their jobs while they were coping with their own stress. One woman said she felt like a leper whenever she left the hospital. Another was teaching a part-time course at the University of Toronto at the time, but when she arrived to give her class, she was asked to leave. Others spoke of being denied dental care for themselves or daycare services for their children.

And for those health care heroes who worked directly with patients who had SARS, they experienced "work quarantine." This meant they were confined to their wards in the hospital, no longer allowed to leave the floor to meet other colleagues for meals in the cafeteria or to go to meetings. And when these brave men and women went home at the end of an exhausting shift, they were quarantined within their houses and from their families. They could not leave their homes to do errands, and, inside their own walls, had to wear masks and eat and sleep alone. As they headed off to their next shifts, they often took with them their neighbors' curses, their partners' anger, and their children's fears that they would get sick and die. As one nurse put it, "It was as hard as it gets!"

Being Together: The Power of Family

Even though the SARS outbreak has been over for two years, the damage lingers. While no one really knows the depth of trauma that still haunts patients and families from that period, many staff will privately admit to suffering from post-traumatic stress. One hospital had a psychiatrist who would meet with the staff most affected every day during the crisis and debrief with them, but staff from another hospital had no support at all—not during the outbreak or since. "We're professionals. We're supposed to be tough. We love what we do and we went into health care to help people. And we learned that we have to help each other at times like this. But the emotional burden of dealing with this is huge." Some quietly express fears about possible future outbreaks of infectious diseases: "I think some staff will just refuse to come to work, and then where will we be?"

For those committed to family-centered care, it has been additionally difficult to hear some of their colleagues say how much they enjoyed not having what they called the "noise and chaos" of having family members around during SARS, that they found it more peaceful to work. As families return to the hallways of these hospitals and staff adjust to the increased traffic, hopefully too will come the reminders that patient recovery, competence, and satisfaction are all increased with the information, support, and presence of families respected for their contributions.

One team of nurses and social workers put it this way: "Certainly SARS showed that in a time of crisis, elements of care we value can be easily lost or destroyed. We are passionate about family-centered care. Even under the best of circumstances, it can be difficult to implement. We have worked long and hard to change the culture of our hospital. The fruits of our labors disappeared overnight, and the road back is proving to be tenuous. The challenge now is for leaders in health care to ensure that policies and systems are in place to allow us to respond to a public health crisis without sacrificing the relationships among patients, families and health care providers."

The word "pandemic" is commonplace in the news of the day, and the world feels somewhat endangered. Consequently, the lessons learned and questions raised by SARS are timely and present a great opportunity for reflection and evaluation. The SARS experience provides an informed basis for planning for the future and, as such, it would be almost unethical to make plans that do not address the emotional side effects of family separation and patient isolation.

In the words of one hospital team, "We need to fully understand the cost/benefit of isolation procedures and find answers to questions such as:

♦ How restrictive do limits on contact between professionals and patients and families need to be?

♦ Might the steady presence of a family member naturally reduce the number of contacts while helping the patient and providing support for overworked staff?

♦ How restrictive does access to the hospital need to be?

♦ How widespread is the need to use protective equipment?

♦ How do we use families as advisors to help us in answering these questions?

♦ What support network needs to be in place for staff and their families?"

A lesson learned from the SARS experience is that there must be proactive planning to provide appropriate support for all

those who are directly affected in such public health emergencies
—from public health officials and health care professionals to
patients and their families. There's no question that the first priority in these situations is to protect the safety of people and control the spread of an outbreak. At the same time, however, it is
also important to find ways not to abandon the standards of family-centered care and to ensure that post-traumatic stress be
averted and/or treated.

Now is the time to plan for "the next infectious disease emergency." It is essential to bring many different points of view to the
table to find the best ways to respond—including public health
and infection control specialists charged with protecting public
safety; patients and family members; hospital leaders; and those
front-line staff who tried their best to deliver compassionate care.
It is only through such an inclusive collaboration that the full
ramifications of the SARS crisis will be addressed, innovative
solutions will be suggested, and responsive systems will be put in
place to sustain and support patients, families, and staff.

---

*Government officials, infection control specialists, public health personnel, hospital leaders, and front-line staff caught in the vortex of
the SARS experience were faced with phenomenal and frightening
uncertainty. They were called upon to demonstrate tremendous
courage, day in and day out. They are to be praised for caring, coping, and finding creative ways to adapt clinical practice in a climate
of such restrictions. Their wish is that others "get ready."*

*This SARS story is the result of many conversations with and
contributions from staff from different Toronto hospitals and infection control specialists in the United States.*

~

It's Not About Time:
Small Moments and Lasting Memories

"When serious illness strikes, each one of us
wants not simply the best possible care for our body
but for our whole being."
—*Kenneth B. Schwartz*

"Watch your thoughts; they become words.
Watch your words; they become actions.
Watch your actions; they become habits.
Watch your habits; they become your character.
Watch your character; it becomes your destiny."
—*Frank Outlaw*

"You may never know what results come from
your action. But if you do nothing,
there will be no result."
—*Gandhi*

~

It's not just what happens, it's also how things happen.
It's not just what you do, but how you are.
It's not simply about techniques, treatments,
and technology; it's also about genuine, authentic,
compassionate communication and relationships.

Think about the impact of . . . a smile . . . a hug . . .
holding a hand . . . seeing past a bandage to look at the
world with a patient's eyes . . . a warm look, a kind
gesture . . . sharing tears . . . the briefest pause in the
frenetic pace of the day . . . as opposed to . . . being left
alone in a time of crisis . . . being callously dismissed at
a time of stress . . . having no one notice your pain or
your tears . . . overhearing disturbing conversations
about you and your prognosis. . . .

EVERYDAY GIFTS
LINGERING EFFECTS
SIMPLE SENTENCES
MAKING THE UNBEARABLE BEARABLE
SHE SANG HIM HIS LIFE
THE MAGIC OF MUSIC
THANKS FOR THE GOOD SEATS
WITHIN A SINGLE DAY

EVERYDAY GIFTS

The Lady in Red

I RECALL GETTING ON THE ELEVATOR AND JOINING A MAN AND A WOMAN. She was wearing a red outfit and a turban under which I could tell she had no hair and was on active therapy. Her face broke into a glorious smile as she said, "Good morning!" As she moved next to me, I realized she was standing behind her husband, hugging his waist, grimacing in severe pain. Yet as she began to exit the elevator, she smiled again and said, "Have a nice day!" She came to the hospital that day with courage, faith, and hope, and her very being was a testament to the strength of the human spirit.

Coaching

Scott was thirty-five and a wrestling coach, diagnosed with colorectal cancer. Two years after surgery and extraordinary health care journeys, he was invited to talk to a group of professionals to provide a patient's view of the discharge process. Later, reflecting on his talk, he said, "I've just done the most important thing in my life. It is such a privilege to help others."

9-11

The day after planes hit the World Trade Center and the Pentagon, our waiting room was full of people needing care. For them, their illnesses were their disasters, and they needed us to function. It was an awesome experience to try to put ourselves in their shoes and get past the news. I was reminded that day of a proverb that says, "He who plants a garden has faith in tomorrow." We were gardeners that day.

―――――――――

These reflections come from a senior hospital administrator who says, "If we just pay attention, our patients give us gifts every day. They are at the center of everything we do."

LINGERING EFFECTS

EVERYTHING FELT NEW. We'd been married for three years and had decided to move to a new city and a new country. We only knew two people when we arrived in May. And then we got pregnant. It was June.

The excitement of having our first child changed to worry when the baby stopped moving. Worry changed to deep sorrow when the doctor told us that the baby was no longer alive in my uterus. He said it would be safest to allow my body to go into labor naturally when it chose to do so. It was September.

When people looked at us and said, "Oh, you're pregnant, dear—how wonderful—when are you due?" we simply smiled meekly and walked away. And we waited.

Things that needed doing were put on hold. But finally my husband had to go and close up our cottage. A couple of hours after he left, in the early evening, I went into labor. It was November.

An old family friend took me to the hospital. When I got there, a doctor examined me. Noticing my anxiety and fear, he glibly said, "Why are you so upset?"

The hospital staff said that they didn't have a bed for me and were going to send me home. My friend was madder than a hornet! I think I would have been completely neglected if she hadn't been there. Sadly, she couldn't stay.

I was alone all night and in labor for nine hours. Then the labor pains stopped. At 6 A.M., I had to go to the bathroom. It didn't seem normal. It felt like I had passed something. I called the nurse. She looked and said, "Oh, it's just a clot." She flushed the toilet.

But it was our baby. I shut down emotionally for years.

Even though this couple went on to have three children, it took them a long time to fully understand the damage done by a single, thoughtless sentence and a single, thoughtless act. Twelve years after this death of their first child, they decided to acknowledge his existence in their lives. They named him Matthew. As a family, with their three children, they built a small box, and each of them put something into the box. Coincidentally, when they picked the day for a memorial service, it turned out to be the Day of the Holy Innocents, and the reading suggested for that day by the church was from the Book of Matthew.

SIMPLE SENTENCES

Egypt?

THE NEWS WAS NOT GOOD. Andrea thought that she had beaten her breast cancer, but the doctor had just finished telling her and her husband that she now had a brain tumor.

Andrea and her husband had been planning a special trip to Egypt. She asked her doctor, "Do you think we can still go?" He answered, "It depends on where you want to die."

———————

Andrea did not go to Egypt but lived for several more months.

The Receptionist's Call

Hilary began to feel sick in midsummer. Her doctor sent her for some tests, and the early results, combined with her symptoms, suggested pancreatic cancer. She was scheduled for a fine-needle biopsy that would provide more detailed information. The procedure turned out to be a terrible experience, because it took three times for the technician to "get enough cells." Hilary said she felt like a beaten-up sack of potatoes by the time it was over.

Hilary knew that the results of the biopsy would determine if the surgeon thought he could operate. She also understood that surgery would really be her only chance for, if not a cure, at least some time. She waited for the doctor to call. And then the phone rang. It was the doctor's receptionist, who simply said, "I'm calling to tell you that the surgeon will not be operating at this time."

Hilary valued every day she had and described every moment she had as precious. She was in her garden two days before she died, two months after the phone call.

Overheard

When my mum was ninety-seven, she was admitted to the hospital with pneumonia. A doctor came into her room to report the results of the X-rays. He presumed that my mother was asleep and spoke directly to me: "The diagnosis isn't good. At that age, they often don't survive."

When the doctor left, the older woman grinned and said to her daughter, "You tell him I'm not dead yet!"

MAKING THE UNBEARABLE
BEARABLE

I HAD SPENT A CONSIDERABLE PART OF MY CAREER AS A HEALTH CARE LAWYER, FIRST IN STATE GOVERNMENT AND THEN IN THE PRIVATE SECTOR. I came to know a lot about health care policy and management, government regulations, and contracts. But I knew little about the delivery of care. All that changed on November 7, 1994, when, at age forty, I was diagnosed with advanced lung cancer. In the months that followed, I was subjected to chemotherapy, radiation, surgery, and news of all kinds—most of it bad. It has been a harrowing experience for me and for my family. And yet, the ordeal has been punctuated by moments of exquisite compassion. I have been the recipient of an extraordinary array of human and humane responses to my plight. These acts of kindness—the simple human touch from my caregivers— have made the unbearable bearable.

During September and October of 1994, I made several visits to the outpatient clinic of a Boston teaching hospital for treatment of a persistent cough, low-grade fever, malaise, and weakness. The nurse practitioner diagnosed me as having atypical pneumonia and prescribed an antibiotic. Despite continued abnormal blood counts, she assured me that I had a post-viral infection and didn't need an appointment with my physician until mid-November, if then. By mid-October, I felt so bad that I decided I could not wait until November 11 to be seen. Disappointed with the inaccessibility of my physician, I decided to seek care elsewhere, with the hope that a new doctor might be more responsive.

It's Not About Time: Small Moments and Lasting Memories

My brother, a physician who had trained at Massachusetts General Hospital (MGH), arranged for an immediate appointment with Dr. Jose Vega, an experienced internist affiliated with the MGH. Dr. Vega spent an hour with me and ordered tests, including a chest X-ray. He called within hours to say he was concerned by the results, which showed a mass in my right lung, and he ordered a computerized tomography scan for more detail. I remember leaving my office for home, saying quickly to my secretary, Sharyn Wallace, "I think I may have a serious medical problem." Indeed, the CT scan confirmed abnormal developments in my right lung and chest nodes.

The next day, Dr. Vega, assuring me that he would continue to be available to me whenever I needed him, referred me to Dr. Thomas Lynch, a thirty-four-year-old MGH oncologist specializing in lung cancer. Dr. Lynch, who seems driven by the ferocity of the disease he sees every day, told me that I had lung cancer, lymphoma, or some rare lung infection, although it was most likely lung cancer.

My family and I were terrified. For the next several months, my blood pressure, which used to be a normal 124 over 78, went to 150 over 100, and my heart rate, which used to be a low 48, ran around 100.

Within seventy-two hours of seeing Dr. Lynch, I was scheduled for a bronchoscopy and a mediastinoscopy—exploratory surgical procedures to confirm whether I indeed had lung cancer. Until this point, I had thought that I was at low risk for cancer: I was relatively young, I did not smoke (although I had smoked about a cigarette a day in college and in law school and for several years after that), I worked out every day, and I avoided fatty foods.

Making the Unbearable Bearable

The day before surgery, I was scheduled to have a series of tests. The presurgical area of the hospital was mobbed, and the nurses seemed harried. Eventually, a nurse who was to conduct a presurgical interview called my name. Already apprehensive, I was breathing hard.

The nurse was cool and brusque, as if I were just another faceless patient. But once the interview began, and I told her that I had just learned that I probably had advanced lung cancer, she softened, took my hand, and asked how I was doing. We talked about my two-year-old son, Ben, and she mentioned that her nephew was named Ben. By the end of our conversation, she was wiping tears from her eyes and saying that while she normally was not on the surgical floor, she would come to see me before the surgery. Sure enough, the following day, while I was waiting to be wheeled into surgery, she came by, held my hand, and, with moist eyes, wished me luck.

This small gesture was powerful; my apprehension gave way to a much-needed moment of calm. Looking back, I realize that in a high volume setting, the high pressure atmosphere tends to stifle a caregiver's inherent compassion and humanity. But the briefest pause in the frenetic pace can bring out the best in a caregiver and do much for a terrified patient.

The nurse left, and my apprehension mounted. An hour later, I was wheeled to surgery for a biopsy of the chest nodes and the mass in my lung. I was greeted by a resident in anesthesiology, Dr. Debra Reich, who took my pulse and blood pressure and said gently, "You're pretty nervous, huh?" She medicated me with tranquilizers, but that did not stop me from asking where she lived, where she had trained, and whether she was married. I jokingly asked her how come she was the only Jewish doctor I had met during my time at MGH. When it turned out that she lived down the street from me and liked the sandwiches at the same corner shop, Virginia's, I felt comforted. She squeezed my shoulder, wished me luck, and wheeled me into surgery.

When I awoke, I was told that I had adenocarcinoma in my right lung and in several chest nodes—in other words, advanced lung cancer. I don't remember a lot about those hours, but I remember Dr. Vega's face with tears in his eyes. I also remember feeling very sad and scared.

A few days later, I received a letter from Dr. Reich:

Remember me, your friendly anesthesiologist? I came by to see you this afternoon as my professional duty but also to express my sadness in hearing about your diagnosis. Your door was closed and there seemed to be a lot of activity, so I decided not to disturb you.

As I'm sure you know, we as physicians are taught not to become emotionally involved in our patients, because then we would be continually devastated. But I guess because we had such a nice interaction before your surgery and because your life was one which I could relate to so well—being Jewish, professional, renovating a house, sandwiches at Virginia's, etc.—your situation really struck a chord in me. (Hey, maybe you can't even remember any of this because of the medicine I gave you, but hopefully you do.)

I was impressed that during the fear and anxiety you were experiencing, you still maintained your composure, your sense of humor, and even thought to ask me when I was getting married.

So anyway, as you told me, keeping your wife and son in mind will make you fight strong, and I know this to be true! I know that you have a very loving and supportive family who will help you through this as well.

Best wishes, and maybe I'll run into you sometime at Virginia's.

I had not forgotten Dr. Reich, nor will I ever forget her willingness to cross the professional barrier, hold my hand, and write those words.

It was clear that I would soon begin a new chapter in my illness and undergo the classic treatment for such advanced cancer: intensive chemotherapy and radiation, followed by surgery to remove the tumors, the nodes, and the entire lung, if necessary. Dr. Lynch told me that this option presented the real possibility of a cure.

Over the next week, I had a series of additional radiologic scans to determine if the cancer had spread beyond my chest. These scans are incredibly scary: You are placed in a tube resembling a sarcophagus, with only six inches between you and the walls, and you may spend several hours inside, deafened by the clanging machine. And the scans always raise fears about whether more bad news is around the corner.

Dr. Vega or Dr. Lynch always made it a point, though, to relay results within twenty-four hours, so my family and I didn't have to endure the anxiety of uncertainty any longer than necessary.

The scans of my body, head, liver, bones, and back were clear. I was relieved.

The doctors soon began an intensive regimen of chemotherapy and radiation, with the goal of destroying the cancer and preparing for surgery to remove my lung.

It's Not About Time: Small Moments and Lasting Memories

Before being admitted for my first five-day course of chemotherapy, I had a radiation-simulation session. During such sessions, therapists meticulously map their targets by marking your skin where the radiation should be directed. I was asked to lie on a table in a large, cold chamber. The radiation therapist, Julie Sullivan, offered me a blanket and, mentioning that the staff had a tape deck, asked if I had any requests. I recalled my college days and asked for James Taylor. Listening to "Sweet Baby James" and "Fire and Rain," I thought back to a time when the most serious problem I faced was being jilted by a girlfriend, and tears ran down my cheeks. As therapists came and went, Julie Sullivan held my hand and asked me if I was okay. I thanked her for her gentleness.

After having a Port-o-Cath implanted in my chest—a device that allows chemotherapy to be administered without constant needle sticks in the arm—I was admitted to MGH in mid-November. During that and other hospitalizations, either my mother or sister would stay overnight, often sleeping in cramped chairs. When I awoke at night in an anxious sweat or nauseated, I would see one of them and feel reassured.

While doctors managed my medical care, my day-to-day quality of life and comfort were in the hands of two or three nurses. These nurses showed competence and pride in their work, but they also took a personal interest in me. It gave me an enormous boost, and while I do not believe that hope and comfort alone can overcome cancer, they certainly made a huge difference to me during my time in the hospital.

During the period between my two chemotherapies, when I also received high-dose radiation twice a day, I came to know a most exceptional caregiver, the outpatient oncology nurse Mimi Bartholomay. An eight-year veteran who had experienced cancer in her own family, she was smart, upbeat, and compassionate. I had to receive fluids intravenously every day at the clinic, and while I was there, we talked regularly about life, cancer, marriage, and children. She, too, was willing to cross that professional Rubicon—to reach out and talk about my fear of dying or, even worse, my fear of not living out my life, of not biking through the hills of Concord and Weston on summer weekends with my brother, of not seeing my child grow up, of not holding my wife in my arms. And she took the risk of talking about her own father's recent bout with cancer. I cannot emphasize enough how meaningful it was to me when caregivers revealed something about themselves that made a personal connection to my plight. It made me feel much less lonely. The rule books, I'm sure, frown on such intimate engagement between caregiver and patient. But maybe it's time to rewrite them.

After my second round of chemotherapy, I was ready for the final stage of what we hoped would be a cure: surgery. Before this could happen, Dr. Lynch repeated my radiologic scans to be sure that the cancer had not spread. He assured me that the chance of any such metastasis was remote—less than 5 percent—although it would be a disaster if it occurred.

The scans were endless, scary, and lonely. While members of my family stayed with me in the waiting rooms, they could not accompany me to the scanning rooms; the experience again was harrowing. But I felt my greatest fear while awaiting the results. After a week of tests, I had one last scan of my bones. I was concerned when the technologist asked to do a special scan of my back that had not been done before.

The next day, I called Dr. Lynch's office and asked his assistant, Mary Ellen Rousell, when I could come in to find out the results. She said, "How about this afternoon?" and then added, "You might want to bring someone." My heart skipped. When my wife and I entered Dr. Lynch's office and saw his face, our hearts sank. He was ashen. He said that while all the other scans were clear, there appeared to be a metastatic tumor in my spine. He explained that this meant that lung surgery at this point would be futile, since other metastases were likely to surface.

Dr. Lynch said that he could not be 100 percent certain that this was a tumor and that, because so much was at stake, we should do a biopsy. My wife and I wept openly—in part, because, looking at Dr. Lynch's face, we felt that he had lost hope.

I could not help but ask what treatment options were available, and he mentioned a drug called Taxol. Still being the lawyer, I quizzed him:

Me: What is the percentage of people who benefit from Taxol?

Dr. Lynch: Forty percent.

Me: How much do they benefit?

Dr. Lynch: They can get several years of life, although it is not a a cure. And the median survival for patients on Taxol with your advanced stage of disease is nine months.

Nine months! My wife and I cringed. I ended the session by asking Dr. Lynch, "How do you do this work?" And he answered, in genuine pain, "By praying that I don't have days like today."

I began to have trouble sleeping, and when I awoke, I was filled with dread and despair. I thought frequently of the observation of Richard Block, the founder of H&R Block, who had survived lung cancer after being told initially that he had only months to live: "I lived for five days without hope and . . . my life during those five days . . . was far worse than at any time during the 'horrible' ordeal of tests and treatments."

And when I contemplated not living to see my son grow up or not cherishing my wife for a lifetime, I thought of King Lear, who, at a low point, wailed:

> I am bound
> Upon a wheel of fire, that mine own tears
> Do scald like molten lead.

A few days later, I had the biopsy. Dr. Lynch met with my family to report that, indeed, after considerable searching, the pathologist had found small deposits of adenocarcinoma in my vertebra. It was now confirmed that I had metastatic lung cancer. Although my brother and my father, who is also a physician, raised the possibility of radical surgery on my back and lung to remove all the tumors, Dr. Lynch and the surgeons rejected this option because further metastases were likely to appear, and the surgery would be debilitating and reduce my quality of life at a time when my life could well be substantially shortened.

The clear treatment was more chemotherapy. Dr. Lynch again recommended the use of Taxol, with the hope of slowing the cancer's spread.

My wife and I were largely silent during the medical discussion. I asked my father and brother to leave so that my wife and I could talk not facts and figures but matters of the heart. When they had left, I said to Dr. Lynch, "You told me two things all along: One, that you were aiming for a total cure, and if that were not feasible, you would tell me at that time. And two, you would never, ever give up on me, never stop trying to fight, to extend my life as long as possible. Am I no longer on the cure route?"

He looked somberly at us and explained that there were no known treatments to cure this stage of cancer.

"And will you stick by me and fight to the end?" I asked.

He nodded vigorously and then outlined a number of state-of-the-art, experimental protocols from which I might benefit after Taxol.

And leaving statistics behind, he talked of several patients who had defied the odds and lived for years beyond expectations. He advised that my goal should be to be here the same time next year, and then the year after, and the year after—one day at a time. He mentioned several breast-cancer patients who had told him that they had relished their final years with their children in a way that they had never known before. It felt good to leave the medical talk and speak heart to heart, and it felt to me that he had regained a sense of hope—not for some magical cure, but for the possibility of extending my life.

It was crucial to my wife and to me that he not give up hope. I understood his surprise and disappointment at the metastases; in fact, as one friend suggested, his distress at that event was a sign of his caring about me and his involvement with my case. But we desperately needed him to give us a realistic basis for hope—and he had.

The next day, I began a new chapter in my fight. And once again, Mimi Bartholomay was by my side, monitoring my reaction and assuring me that most people tolerated Taxol very well. I had no allergic reaction, and I felt good that the battle was underway. I had hoped that maybe this could buy me time.

Time was now my best friend, since it could allow medical research to advance and doctors to find new strategies and maybe even a cure for advanced lung cancer.

Making the Unbearable Bearable

During this period, with help from my father, who has had a long and distinguished career in academic medicine, I began to explore potential cutting-edge protocols that could supplement or follow Taxol.

My father arranged a meeting for my wife and me with Dr. Kurt J. Isselbacher, a distinguished researcher and director of the MGH Cancer Center. He is a small man with a large presence and piercing blue eyes, and he was surrounded by medical books, papers, and many pictures of his family. He was upbeat, telling us of protocols underway that showed promise in fighting metastatic tumors. Like several others, he told me a personal story that cut to the bone: A close family member, he said, had been diagnosed with advanced cancer, which the attending oncologist had said was "very, very bad." The family member had said to him, "Kurt, you have helped so many people in your life; can you now help me?" He personally treated the family member in that person's home with chemotherapy, and, twenty-one years later, that person is thriving.

Dr. Isselbacher offered to serve as an advocate for me, to work with my father and Dr. Lynch to find the most promising protocols. I told him at the meeting that while I had no illusions, I was deeply moved by his refusal to give up and by his abiding hope. I was especially affected because such hopefulness was not coming from a faith healer, but from a distinguished researcher. He had strengthened our resolve to fight.

As I grappled to maintain my hope in the face of the advancing disease, I was referred to Dr. Ned Cassem, a senior MGH psychiatrist who not only had had vast experience with the seriously ill, but was himself a Jesuit priest. I had met with him once during my second hospitalization, and my memory through the haze was that he was the first person with whom I had discussed death. I remembered that when I asked him if, when, and how I should say goodbye to people, he said, "You know, you don't have to wait to say goodbye; you can express your love and appreciation for people right now, every day."

After the devastating news of the metastases, I felt the urge to seek out Dr. Cassem again, in part to ask if there was anything more I should be doing to help my son, Ben, cope with my illness or the eventuality of my death. I mentioned that several people had suggested I make a videotape for Ben, but I thought I couldn't do that. Dr. Cassem replied that every time we played or laughed together, we were creating building blocks, precious memories that will be a part of him forever.

I also asked him if he thought I should be doing more to prepare for the possibility of an early death. He looked perplexed and asked, "Have you prepared your will?" I said yes. "Are your affairs otherwise in order?" I again said yes. "So it sounds like you are prepared. Remember, death is a minor matter. Living . . . that's the challenge."

I then told him of the paradox that moments of great pleasure—playing with my son, snuggling with my wife, talking intensely with friends—also caused me great pain and tears. Was I depressed? Was this something to worry about? He looked at me thoughtfully and said, "When you cry about your son, it's because he has touched you deeply. It's an affirmation of your love for him. When you weep about the joy you experienced with your wife or close friends, that's an acknowledgment of your love for them. That's not a bad thing. Maybe a day without tears has been a dull day." I nodded and then could not help but ask, "Do you believe in the power of prayer?" Dr. Cassem nodded. "Absolutely," he said, "and your name is on my prayer list." I felt warmed in his presence, by his wisdom, his common sense, and his spirituality.

In recent months, I have had several setbacks: a bone scan that showed four to five additional tumors, and a CT scan that showed significant progression of the cancer in both lungs. The only good news was that it had not spread to my head or liver. I am pained, but not surprised, at the relentlessness of the disease, and I am straining to retain hope that one of the experimental treatments may succeed where chemotherapy has failed.

For the first time, I recently mentioned to Dr. Lynch the idea of a hospice service and wondered how I might reduce future pain as the cancer progresses. Dr. Lynch answered that we were still a long way from that discussion, that we still had many avenues to explore, and that he remained as committed as ever to doing whatever he could to extend my life in a quality way.

Around the time of the CT scan, when I was feeling particularly dejected, I had an appointment with Mimi Bartholomay for an injection. She was running late, and as she approached me in the clinic, she looked harried. But as she got closer, she could see how unhappy I was, and she put her arm around me and directed me to a private room. I began to cry, and she intuitively responded, "You know, scan days are the worst. But whatever the results, we are not going to give up on you. We're going to fight with you and for you all the way." I hugged her and thanked her for hanging in there with me.

If I have learned anything, it is that we never know when, how, or whom a serious illness will strike. If and when it does, each one of us wants not simply the best possible care for our body, but for our whole being.

I am still bound upon Lear's wheel of fire, but the love and devotion of my family and friends, and the deep caring and engagement of my caregivers, have been a tonic for my soul and have helped to take some of the sting from my scalding scars.

In my new role as a patient, I have learned that medicine is not merely about performing tests or surgeries, or administering drugs. These functions, important as they are, are just the beginning. For as skilled and knowledgeable as my caregivers are, what matters the most is that they have empathized with me in a way that gives me hope and makes me feel like a human being, not just an illness.

Again and again, I have been touched by the smallest kind gestures—a squeeze of my hand, a gentle touch, a reassuring word. In some ways, these quiet acts of humanity have felt more healing than the high-dose radiation and chemotherapy that hold the hope of a cure.

As an eminent Harvard Medical School professor, himself a cancer patient, once taught, "The secret of the care of the patient is caring for the patient."

Kenneth B. Schwartz died of lung cancer in September 1995. Shortly before his death, he founded The Kenneth B. Schwartz Center (see page 263) at Massachusetts General Hospital, which is dedicated to strengthening the relationship between patients and caregivers.

This story, by Kenneth B. Schwartz, originally appeared in The Boston Globe Magazine *on July 16, 1995, under the title "A Patient's Story." With minor changes to reflect the passage of time, it is reprinted here with the permission of The Kenneth B. Schwartz Center.*

SHE SANG HIM HIS LIFE

PALLIATIVE CARE SEEMS TO BE A PLACE WHERE ANYTHING GOES. On our unit, the hours are completely open; people come and go as they need; pets visit. Staff pay attention to so many little details of comfort. There's a tenderness and kindness on the unit that's extraordinary. By comparison, when I visit someone on another floor, it's impersonal, and I feel assaulted by noise, unpleasant smells, and a sense of crowdedness.

One night, I arrived for my regular volunteer shift on the palliative care unit and found the staff in a very emotional state. This was not entirely unusual, but I sensed that something special had happened that day. I was right.

A young man, in his early forties, had been on the unit for several days. His wife had been with him almost constantly. This husband and wife were both from the same tiny village in Newfoundland. They had grown up together, become a couple, gotten married, and lived there all their lives. And now this man, her husband, was dying.

She knew that the end was near and asked the nurses if she could get into bed with her husband and snuggle. And the answer was, "Of course you can, dear."

And then the singing started. It went on for well over an hour. This woman, as she cuddled her dying husband, slowly and gently, sang him his life and their lives together.

When the singing stopped, her husband was still alive. She then she sang him permission to leave.

When asked why this woman chose to become a volunteer in palliative care, she explained that it was because of her experience with her father. When he was dying, in a different hospital and far away, she says that the care he received in palliative care was so dear that she told herself, "This is what I'm going to do some day."

THE MAGIC OF MUSIC

MUSIC FOR ME IS LIKE MAGIC. When I go to the extendicare center where I work part-time, what I see when I walk in are so many old people, sitting in wheelchairs. They are not doing anything, not saying anything, not noticing anyone or anything around them. But then I start to play and sing songs from the 1920s and 1930s. Toes begin tapping, then I hear a gentle humming followed by tentative words, and soon, the whole room has come alive. People sing and talk to each other, sharing stories about memories evoked by the music.

Staff participate as well. The music appears to be therapy for them, too. They seem more excited about the work they're doing and the people they're working with. They see that behind the usual blank stares, there are people with rich past lives.

There's one woman I work with on a one-to-one basis, because she has a bad back and it's hard for her to sit. When I go in to see her, she's usually sprawled across her bed, dozing. I gently nudge her awake and she gets very excited. I play songs like "Frankie and Johnny" and "Five Foot Two" for her, because she knows all the words and sings right along. She sits right up and waves her arms in rhythm with the music. When I have to leave, she always says, "Please don't go. Please don't go." I feel guilty, because there's generally a lethargic feeling in the air and not much incentive to be active or intellectually stimulated.

I also work on a psychiatric unit with people from ages eighteen to eighty. My goal is to provide a joyful and magical experience for everyone through music making and improvisation. Music is a great vehicle for socializing and having a good time, breaking down age barriers, and providing some positive distraction from worries. Two particular experiences stand out in my mind.

One night, I remember singing James Taylor's "Fire and Rain," which has the words "I always knew I'd see you again" in reference to someone who has died. One of the women who was in the hospital for depression started to cry. It turned out that her husband had recently died. She thanked me, saying that crying felt like a great release. She then asked if she could have a copy of the words. When I returned, I brought her a copy of the lyrics. She was so surprised and delighted that I had remembered.

Another time, a cluster of young patients in their twenties, very much part of the rave scene, asked me to bring in some progressive house and trance music. When I did, the young kids started dancing while the other patients watched in awe. Eventually, everyone, even the patients in their seventies, started dancing. The young people felt very positive about having contributed something enjoyable to others on the unit, and they remarked they'd had a good time. They didn't know it was possible to do so without drugs and alcohol.

It's exciting to see music helping people progress and improve. It is interesting to me that attendance on the nights when Music with Ann is offered is about 80 percent, whereas attendance for activities such as crafts, games, and outings is only 30 percent.

Tragically, music is often seen as a frill, and music therapy is usually at the bottom of the budget pile. But I'll keep writing proposals, because I see the magic that happens with music.

––––––––––––

Ann is a certified music therapist. Her dream job would be to work in psychiatry full-time.

THANKS FOR THE GOOD SEATS

WE HAD A GENTLEMAN ON OUR UNIT WHO HAD CANCER OF THE BRAIN.
One night, when he seemed particularly restless, I suggested that
we go to the cafeteria for tea. Ever the gentleman, he seemed
worried and said, "But I don't have any money." I told him not to
worry about that.

Try to picture the scene. He has a huge bandage on his head
and is wearing hospital pajamas. I'm in street clothes. Once I got
him comfortable in his wheelchair, the two of us set off.

It was nighttime, and there was an enormous blizzard blowing outside. The cafeteria has huge glass windows to the outside.
Because it was dark outside and the cafeteria lights were on, these
windows reflected the room. However, the reflection was not
complete, like a mirror, because you could still see the storm and
the twinkling lights of the snowy parking lot.

I wasn't really paying attention to any of this as I settled my
gentleman at a table. We chatted briefly about what kind of a
doughnut he would like as a special treat, and I said I'd be right
back. When I returned with his tea and doughnut, he looked up
at me and said, "Thanks for getting us such good seats for the
show." I suddenly got it—I got under his bandage and saw the
world with his eyes—and, stifling my laughter, I simply said,
"You're welcome."

WITHIN A SINGLE DAY

WITHIN A SINGLE DAY, I SAW SOME OF THE BEST AND THE WORST OF CURRENT PRACTICE. My mother-in-law and I were accompanying my father-in-law to consultations with two different pulmonary oncologists. For the first visit, the three of us were taken into a room with four stretchers and only curtains for privacy. My eighty-year-old father-in-law was asked to sit on the edge of a stretcher with his legs dangling over the side. There was a chair for my mother-in-law; I stood.

When the doctor finally arrived, he did not acknowledge my mother-in-law or me. He spoke directly to my father-in-law, saying, "I talk quietly, so you will have to turn up your hearing aid." With barely a pause, he continued saying, "I've looked at the test results. You have a cancer that won't respond to treatment. There's nothing we can do for you."

He basically left us with no hope. He conveyed no feelings or concern for our experience. He failed to provide any information about what would happen. He offered no help for how we would manage in the coming days and weeks. He didn't ask us if we had any questions. It was as though my father-in-law was merely an irritating, negative test result in his busy day. The doctor walked out, leaving the three of us there alone and stunned. Although he said nothing, my father-in-law's stooped shoulders and hanging head communicated complete despair.

The afternoon encounter was another story altogether. The second doctor invited the three of us into a room with comfortable chairs, asked everyone to sit, and spoke to each of us by name, making sure he understood how we were all connected to my father-in-law. In essence, he had the same message as the morning doctor, but he delivered it so differently. He was clear about there being no further curative interventions, but was also clear about saying, "I want to work together with you. How can I be most helpful?" He answered our questions and engaged us all in discussion. We did not feel alone and, even better, we felt we were part of a team.

I was struck by the difference between these two experiences in the same day. While the diagnosis was still awful, there was a sense of caring and compassion offered by the afternoon doctor that made us feel supported and encouraged us to believe that we could cope. We often hear that there's no time for compassion in health care, but both of these encounters took exactly the same amount of time!

The day reinforced my belief that health care is about people, about communication and relationships, and about helping patients and families deal with difficult situations. It's not just about whether a professional can fix or not fix something.

~

Hope for the Future:
Passion for the Possible

"Determine the thing that is to be done
and then we will find the way."
—*Abraham Lincoln*

"We are such stuff as dreams are made of . . ."
—*William Shakespeare*

"We are not in a position in which we have
nothing to work with. We already have capacities,
talent, direction, missions, callings."
—*Abraham Maslow*

"Risk more than others think is safe.
Care more than others think is wise.
Dream more than others think is practical.
Expect more than others think is possible."
—*Cadet Maxim, U.S. Military Academy, West Point*

"We are all waiting for an invitation to do good."
—*Gerri Frager, M.D.*

~

Hope for the future of patient- and family-centered
health care is embedded in two sentinel facts:
first, that any number of examples already exist of the
kind of care we all hope to have . . . care that is
compassionate, collaborative, and based on dignity,
respect, and full, transparent communication;
and second, that there are people working hard to make
change and to maintain gains that have been made.

Just as the legendary phoenix rises from ashes,
often from a situation of great challenge comes
something good.

LEARNING FROM TRAGEDY
THE CAPACITY TO DO GOOD
FINDING MEANING IN CHAOS
IT DOESN'T TAKE MUCH
THE WHITE COAT
WHEN THE WORLD TURNS UPSIDE DOWN
CREATING A CULTURE

LEARNING FROM TRAGEDY

I joined Dana-Farber Cancer Institute (DFCI) in 1995, six months after a tragic and much publicized medication error led to the untimely death of a cancer patient who was also a well-known health columnist for the *Boston Globe*. Staff were anxious, apprehensive, insecure, and grieving. They knew we had to deliver care and were committed to that, yet they also knew everyone was looking at us and "wondering."

At the time, I believed we had a responsibility to learn everything we could about the causes of the medication error, to take steps to make sure such a mistake never happened again, then to turn the tragedy into a vision and practice of being the very best place to receive cancer care. As part of this process, we realized we needed to speak openly and honestly about what had happened and what we were going to do about it. In the first two years after the tragedy, we spoke to thousands of leaders across the country via a series of Joint Commission on Accreditation of Healthcare Organizations (JCAHO) presentations as well as many others. The support of the organization and the interest in our journey was rewarding and invigorating.

We had many areas of key learning and change in response to the tragedy. Some of the biggest changes were made around involving patients and families. I had come to DFCI from a children's hospital, where we were used to working with patients and families all the time. Yet, when I moved into adult care, I couldn't find the patients or families anywhere except in patient rooms.

I used to tell staff at DFCI that, in pediatrics, we had already learned that "there's no stronger force in the world than a parent in your face!" We also had learned how much patients and families have to offer.

Hope for the Future: Passion for the Possible

I wanted to put patients and families at the center of our world. I engaged the board and key patient care leaders. We started by just listening to patients and their families and inviting them into a few processes. Many staff thought this was crazy, but within weeks they were saying, "They're teaching us things we didn't know." Within the first year, we had more than 100 patients and family members on committees.

Now we involve patients, family members, and survivors on virtually every clinical operations committee in the hospital, including search committees for senior staff, employee orientation programs, construction programs, and the quality improvement and risk management committee of the board. The involvement of patients and families has become an expectation, not an exception. I am convinced this has led to better, safer, and more respectful and compassionate clinical care and success.

There is now a profound awareness of the unique insights and advice that those who have been the recipients of care can bring to the table. Their observations and suggestions have led to a wide variety of changes that include structural improvements in renovation projects, a new fast-track system for immuncompromised patients arriving in pediatric emergency, a patient rounding program by patients and family members, supportive therapies such as massage and acupuncture, and a program in which patients teach physicians-in-training how to break bad news and how to stay connected to and ensure support for patients and families when clinical therapies have run their course. We have even cracked the hard nut of reducing waiting times in clinics and have sought their assistance in billing notices.

I believe that involving patients and families raises the quality of care and reinforces the notion of a partnership in care as suggested by the expression, "Nothing about me, without me." We need to be alerted to problems in real time, rather than having to wait for patient satisfaction surveys to be tabulated and summarized. We also need to design procedures and facilities to meet the needs of patients and families. Only they can tell us what those needs are.

For example, one day I got a call from one of our patients about the overcrowded conditions in our infusion area. I went down and met with the nurse manager, patients, and family members. Everyone agreed that the lack of patient privacy and nursing work space was unacceptable. Existing plans to renovate the unit were halted, and patients and staff gathered to reassess them. The end result is an area that is now much more respectful of and comfortable for all. I have no idea how many people that patient helped with his single phone call.

We want to make sure we are improving the right things. And we can only do this by having patients and families with us every step of the way. They remind us that we may be excellent, but we're not perfect yet!

We are blessed to have the commitment of so many people who are both wise and willing to donate their time. One of our hundreds of volunteers, Regina Mead, a former patient and employee of IBM, and now Co-Chair Emeritus of Dana-Farber's Adult Patient and Family Advisory Committee, has said, "When I underwent treatment here, it was obvious it is about the most patient-centered organization I have ever been associated with. From the top administrators to the parking lot attendants—they are all focused on one question: What can I do to make things better for the patient? That's the kind of place I wanted to continue to be associated with."

Have patients and families given us a hard time? Yes. Have they told us things we sometimes didn't want to hear? Yes. But do they feel respected by the organization and feel heard? Yes. And have they created the impetus and provided the perspective to make this a better place? Yes . . . without a doubt!

James B. Conway was Executive Senior Vice-President and Chief Operations Officer at Dana-Farber Cancer Institute. He is now Senior Fellow at the Institute for Healthcare Improvement and Senior Consultant to DFCI.

THE CAPACITY TO DO GOOD

Dr. Gerri Frager, Medical Director of Pediatric Palliative Care at the IWK Health Centre, crossed the courtyard. There was energy in her step. She had said she'd be wearing red shoes. Looking up from her shoes to her face, I noted her smile and felt her warmth. We found a quiet place to talk.

Q. HOW DID YOU BECOME INTERESTED IN PALLIATIVE CARE?

A. It was really several patients I cared for, first as a nurse and later during my internal medicine internship, who helped me understand how important this aspect of care can be. Within the first month of my internship, I knew internal medicine was not for me, and I ultimately switched to pediatrics. While doing a fellowship at Sloan Kettering in New York, I became involved in the Death in America Project, an initiative funded by George Soros to "develop innovative programs in clinical care, research, education, and advocacy to improve the care of the dying." It was an opportunity of a lifetime. Not only did I get to do my own work, I ultimately became part of a network of eighty-seven others who were doing inspiring work.

Q. What does the term "palliative care" mean to you?

A. Comfort, pain management, symptom management, emotional and spiritual support.

Q. You didn't mention death or dying or end of life.

A. I don't think palliative care should just be available to those
    who are dying. There are times when a patient and family
    may need the elements of palliative care—comfort, pain
    management, symptom management—throughout an illness
    that will end in recovery. One shouldn't have to wait until the
    end of life to access this kind of care.

Q. You are the head of a palliative care "service," rather than a
    "unit." What is the difference?

A. I specifically didn't want to have a palliative care unit at this
    hospital for a number of reasons. The most important reason
    is that I think the approaches of palliative care should be
    available everywhere in the hospital and at all times. In this
    hospital, staff are already very sensitive. They provide com-
    petent, compassionate care and collaborate well with fami-
    lies. I don't want to be another layer. I want to work along-
    side others and be a resource to them.

    My job is to help them in their jobs, to provide guidance
    and support when they come up against a new situation in
    which they are not quite sure what to do next. As well, for
    the children and families who come to our health center, and
    particularly for those who have chronic illnesses and come
    repeatedly throughout their lives, they already know the staff
    on their regular units. It would be counterproductive to dis-
    place children and families from those support networks and
    move them to a new, unfamiliar environment, especially one
    with a potentially "loaded" title.

    If someone is in the last days or hours of his or her life, and
    we need more space for extended family and more privacy, we

can take over a couple of rooms and create a sense of quiet on the unit where the patient and family already know the staff and their way around.

Q. How do you support staff?

A. They tell me and our team what they need. I can make clinical suggestions for how the management of pain and other symptoms can be improved. If they want me to do so, I will meet with patients and families, but this is never to take away their role but rather to support their work. Because this is a regional referral hospital, we also consult with staff throughout the region and in remote communities. Sometimes there are "telehealth" conferences with a child's whole care team in that community.

I also listen. People often forget that when a child and family are suffering, the staff suffer too, or when a child dies, the staff grieve, although in obviously very different ways and dimensions than the family. We send bereavement baskets to the unit when a child dies. The baskets contain food, quotes, pictures, candles, little gestures of comfort, and always a card affirming the work they did and acknowledging that it is tough to be the people helping at such a special time in the life of a family.

These baskets are even sent to the outlying communities when we know that a child has died. The first time we did this, we heard, "No one has ever done something like this or thanked us before!"

This next thing may sound simple and small, but I've been surprised by the feedback. I love taking pictures, and I also love quotes and books. I have a bulletin board outside my office, and I pick a theme every couple of months. I put together photos and quotes and make copies available for people to take away. Often people leave notes of thanks or stories about what the picture means to them. Sometimes, I get new pictures and quotes back. It's about comfort and connection and communicating on a different level.

Q. If you could provide advice to young doctors, what would you say?

A. I would tell them that we have the capacity to do good, even when things are not going well, and not to be afraid of being a part of those situations.

Q. Where do your compassion and kindness come from?

A. I believe we all have this inherently in us. Someone once said we are all waiting for an invitation to do good. Sometimes it takes a personal experience to wake up this goodness. Sometimes it takes a special invitation, a specific request.

Q. Can compassion and kindness be learned?

A. Yes. Some people just need help and encouragement to see what they can do. There are some who test my belief, though. At times, you might have to be strategic and creative in how or when you put out the invitation to do good.

And there are some "sharks" out there who seem to be set only on destruction. It's good to be aware of sharks, but I don't want to live my life in fear of them, always looking over my shoulder. I don't want to lose my vulnerability, my soft "underbelly."

Q. From what you know about hospitals, what would you want if you were a patient?

A. I'd want my basic needs of warmth, shelter, and nourishment covered. I'd want to be comfortable enough to see out a window that opens so that I could breathe the air and look out at nature. I'd want some privacy and the capacity to fill my space with the people and a few small things that are meaningful to me.

Q. You provide so much support for others. Who supports you?

A. I make sure I get time to be outdoors, hiking, breathing fresh air, listening to birds, looking at flowers, taking pictures, and sometimes sharing that with someone close to me. Nature nourishes and restores me. I can remember a time, though, when I was involved in the care of two teenagers, back to back, whose dying was protracted, and their diseases completely challenged their independence in terrible ways.

When the second young person died, I was physically exhausted and ravaged by the emotional impact of caring for them. The injustice of their deaths felt so profound. I knew I had to get away.

I spent part of my time away, out in nature. Then I attended a week-long retreat called "Healing the Wounded Healer." It was comforting to be in the presence of others who were also feeling so human and so vulnerable. And now I'm back.

Hope for the Future: Passion for the Possible

Dr. Frager is interested in integrating the arts and health care. She intends to initiate a program for all hospital staff— janitors and laundry workers to doctors and administrators— in which they will take photographs and write about them. When that is done, she wants to offer a similar program for patients and families.

FINDING MEANING IN CHAOS

LINDA CLARKE HAS A VERY LONG TITLE. In addition to being a writer and storyteller, she is the Facilitator of the Program in Narrative Medicine in the Medical Humanities Program of the Faculty of Medicine at Dalhousie University in Halifax, Nova Scotia. Long as the title is, though, it only hints at what she does or why she does it.

In short, Linda is trying to touch the next generation of doctors and open their minds and hearts to the power of hearing and telling stories. She passionately believes that we never feel more validated than when we are invited to share something about ourselves. Stories provide meaning, make connections, and create a sense of community—of belonging.

Linda's journey to this work is an interesting story in itself. Many factors forged Linda's passion for storytelling. It's not as simple as just understanding that she has a background in theater and training in storytelling. It's more personal than that.

Linda's work in health care began in the world of academic bioethics. While she appreciated that the field was principle-driven and designed to be thoughtful and impartial, she longed to get closer to the real people and the real experiences from which ethical issues and questions were arising. This began to happen when Linda moved from a university setting to working directly in a hospital-based clinical ethics service. Working with members of the hospital community, walking the halls, catching conversations over coffee, observing and listening to the caregivers, and, in time, from her own experiences as a patient and the child of a sick father, she witnessed the power of stories firsthand.

"People are the markers of our health care institutions, and stories are the markers of people. We can't respond completely to one another from a distance. Stories are one of the ways we can enter into relationships with one another, and it is from within those relationships that we can provide good care. It is a fundamental act of caring to invite and to receive the story of another person."

Linda continues, "My father had a stroke and lost his speech. I would travel every weekend to be with him and help him navigate the health care system. It was stressful and exhausting. One Monday, when I got back to work, I heard some staff talking about dealing with a difficult family over the weekend. I wondered if they knew anything about the context of that family. I gently interjected to tell them my story. I started with, 'Let me tell you what it may be like to be in their shoes . . .'"

Linda also frames her own experience as a patient in terms of story. When seeking a diagnosis, Linda struggled to have her story of troubling symptoms fully heard by doctors. "As so often happens in the culture of medicine, instead of being able to hear my story in my own terms, doctors would frame what I said within their own world view. 'Headaches? Well, you must be under stress. Fatigue? You're obviously working too hard.'

"My medical story was continuously returned to me, in ways that made sense to the doctors but did not make sense to me. Instead of working with my story, many sent me away, believing their own. I was being required to fit their stories, not the other way around. This is a classic move in the health care culture, but it can feel profoundly dismissive to the person who is ill and seeking care."

Sadly, in spite of months of specific head-related complaints, persistently and eloquently described, a cyst kept growing in the middle of Linda's brain, undiagnosed. It took a crisis before her story was fully heard and believed. "What's really frightening is that I was someone who worked in the hospital. I knew people.

I knew the ropes. If I couldn't get my story heard, what happens to those who are more vulnerable—the elderly, the homeless, people from other cultures, people who do not speak English? How do we hear their stories?"

In her current role, Linda invites medical students to share stories with each other from their own lives. "They don't have to be clever. The medical humanities program, which my work is part of, is not only about creativity. It's about building a context for understanding both yourself and your patients and your community."

Through work with story, students experience firsthand that asking for people's stories makes them feel valued in their entirety. They hear, in their own stories and in the stories of others, not only what happened, but also what was important. Stories help them get to know each other on a different level, and students start to think about what asking for and listening to patients' stories can do for the caregiving relationship.

What unspoken stories can they observe when they go into a patient's room? Is anyone else there—a family member, a friend? Are there cards, photographs? Do they see any books or magazines, and, if so, which ones? Are there bits of food around, and, if so, what? Healthy snacks or junk food? Is the patient listening to music, and, if so, is it classical, jazz, country, or heavy metal?

What can all these little details tell them about the person in the bed? By paying attention and taking cues from the environment, medical students are engaging in eye and ear training for what is to be learned beyond the patient's "principle complaint" and typical charted information. They learn that each clinical case is embodied in a real person who lives his or her particular story in a totally unique fashion.

From noticing, the students move on to asking questions. If they see a photograph on a patient's nightstand, they say, "Tell me who's in your picture." Showing interest in the whole person is an act of shared humanity. A simple question is an invitation to tell a story, and they discover that little details are the doorways to larger stories and to building relationships.

Linda explains:

> The world of patients and families is frightening territory, often rooted in fear of the unknown and loss of meaning, independence, and integrity. Recounting the events of an illness or injury in a story eases these feelings and is often the beginning of healing.
>
> Susan Sontag once said that when you are ill, it's like being in a foreign kingdom. Asking for stories is a bridge back from exile, a place of refuge when all else feels strange, and an important route to insight, compassion, empathy, connection, community. Joan Didion said, "We tell ourselves stories to live."
>
> Health care professionals, too, have stories to tell. These men and women keep company with the suffering of others and walk with them through profound events. The world of health care professionals is full of long hours, pressured situations, hard work, miracles, and tragedies. It can be a raw place with its own pain, fear of the unknown, and loss of meaning. For health care professionals, too, then, telling their stories helps provide comfort and healing for the dramatic work they do. For all, telling stories helps provide meaning in chaos.

IT DOESN'T TAKE MUCH

I'M A THIRD-YEAR MEDICAL STUDENT, A POSITION THAT GRANTS ME THE TITLE OF "CLERK," and I have just finished my first three-month rotation. The word in med school is that your clerkship year is a year of feeling dumb. You're working in hospitals and clinics, and you're wearing a white coat, and people think you're a real doctor. But even with two years of medical school under your belt, all you can think about is how huge and vast is the knowledge you don't yet have!

As humbling as this is, the good news is that, in these first three months, I've learned that while I may not feel smart, I can still contribute to someone's care. I can, with my words and actions, reassure people, provide comfort and support, and listen and not judge. I can make someone's scary time not so scary. While the real professionals are making the big decisions, I have learned that I'm not worthless. I have qualities and abilities that can genuinely help people. It doesn't take much.

For example, just last week, a thirty-five-year-old woman was in the gynecology clinic for a colposcopy. She'd had precancerous lesions on her cervix, and this procedure would remove them. It was my first day in this clinic and everything was new. For the doctor, though, this was going to be his seventeenth procedure of the day—something that would be performed quickly, taking only fifteen minutes.

The patient had her legs up in the air, supported by footrests—the most vulnerable position in the world for a woman. The doctor started the procedure. He is a nice man, but he is "efficient" and doesn't say much as he goes about his work. Sensing this woman's fear and her discomfort, I did what I could to help, squeezing her hand in encouragement and saying things like, "You're doing great," and, "You're almost done."

I ran into this woman when she was leaving the clinic. She said, "I'm so glad you were with me. I know the doctor is an excellent surgeon, but his manner terrifies me. Your being there made it so much less awful."

Another woman was referred to the gynecology clinic for an investigation of persistent, heavy bleeding. She had refused a pelvic examination by her own family doctor, a male, and had waited a potentially life-threatening two years in order to see the female gynecologist of the clinic. Upon reading this information in the referral note, the female doctor was enraged that the referral had been made on the basis of gender. During her first introduction to this patient, she sternly explained that the patient was attending a teaching clinic where the students could very well be male, and she would have to allow their participation, regardless of gender, if she wanted to be seen.

Fortunately for the patient, I was the student that day—a female. After I had taken her history, but before the examination, I presented her case to the doctor, in private. I mentioned that the woman was taking antidepressants and realized I had not determined the reason for this. The doctor asked me to get more information.

When I went back in to see the patient, she was lying on the examining table. I gently explained that I had forgotten to ask her why she was taking antidepressants. She completely broke down and started sobbing. The worry over her gynecological condition was not this patient's only source of stress. She revealed that she was going through a divorce and was not coping. Trembling in the examination room, she seemed so sad and fragile. I covered her with a blanket, sat her up, and did what I could to soothe her. I asked her questions about her children, which calmed her and seemed to strengthen her spirits.

I reported all this to the doctor. When she came in to do the exam, she was not as brusque as she had been before. I continued to hold the woman's hand through the rest of the consult. She was so scared. There was so much going on in her life that she couldn't control.

I spoke to the senior resident about this patient later in the day. She said to me, "You were more of a doctor today than you've ever been. We can have a profound impact on people and can relieve so much suffering with communication and compassion."

On another day, a thirty-two-year-old woman and her husband came in because she was having a miscarriage and needed medical help. Even though miscarriages are relatively common, occurring in approximately 40 percent of medically detectable pregnancies within the first trimester (twelve weeks), this couple had been celebrating their first pregnancy, and they were devastated that it was ending. The attending physician actually asked me to stand by the woman's head to comfort her. I felt the doctor was appreciating that I could play an important role in the care of this couple. He sensed that his knowledge and skill weren't all that was needed in this situation—that empathy was important, too. With some doctors, I feel as though they and I have very different agendas; this day, I felt we were on the same page.

I'm learning so much this year. Of course, I'm learning lots of about medical science and treatment techniques, but I'm also learning that the doctors I appreciate the most are those who know an enormous amount but who still take the time to explain things, in simple language, to their patients. I've observed that two different doctors can spend the same period of twelve minutes with a patient, but one patient will feel like it's been thirty minutes and the other will feel like everything is rushed.

It's such an art to validate someone's concerns, to listen, to ask questions, and to make the patient feel like he or she is playing an important role in the interaction. Words and body language are so important when people are feeling vulnerable.

It's an incredible privilege to be part of someone's health care and their well-being. I'm so grateful I can play a role. People look at you in a white coat, and you become "the trusted one." It's an amazing responsibility and one that I take very seriously. As a clerk, I may often feel dumb with regard to my medical knowledge, but I can be "smart" with regard to compassion. It doesn't take much, but it often makes all the difference in the world.

THE WHITE COAT

EVERY EARLY MORNING, THE SURGEONS, TRAILING A GAGGLE OF MEDICAL
STUDENTS, CLERKS, AND RESIDENTS, MAKE THEIR ROUNDS THROUGH THE
INTENSIVE CARE UNIT (ICU). The group travels from patient to
patient—beds full of them. I could easily picture Mark in that
herd. He was tall and graceful and, no doubt, fresh and bright
even in the early morning: neat white coat, stethoscope nestled
in the pocket, notebook and pen at the ready. Ambitious, smart,
compassionate, and heartful. Every early morning.

A few days into his ICU rotation, Mark noticed that the group
always passed by one patient, a woman in the corner bed. He
began to wonder why she was never included in rounds and it
started to bother him. So one afternoon, when the unit was quiet,
Mark found the time to go to check on her. He was allowed to do
that, with the white coat and the look of authority he was just
then learning to wear comfortably. He found her mostly still,
heavily drugged against pain. Standing quietly at the foot of her
bed, he reviewed her chart: a tumor, growing deep in her brain,
was killing her.

Sitting in my office a few days later, Mark told me about it.
The two of us had made an arrangement some months before
when Mark had first come by to talk about issues concerning
informed consent. One of my roles in the clinical ethics service
was to help students like him work through difficult issues they
were learning to face as they became doctors. Since that time, he
had come by the office every once in awhile to tell me stories
from his practice. It seemed to help him to talk about things, and
it certainly helped me to gain some understanding of the evolu-
tion of a medical practitioner. Snapshots.

And now this.

After reviewing the woman's chart, Mark had spoken with one of the nurses who was looking after the patient.

"She'll die soon," the nurse told him. "Shame she'll die alone."

In my office, the young man stretched out his long legs and looked out the window behind me. He fiddled with the name tag pinned to his white coat, folded neatly in his lap.

"The patient is undocumented," he explained. "No papers that they could find. No health coverage. No status." A pause. "And alone."

I know this happens, even in Canada, once in awhile—people fall through the cracks, especially if they have no home, no address. Or if they land here illegally. Sometimes they don't know how to get health insurance. Even here.

"Well," Mark continued, "she gets good care and everything. It's just that there isn't anyone there to pay"—he paused, searching for the right word—"particular attention to her. No one there just for her."

He fell silent for a moment.

"So I decided I'd try to find out if there was anyone around for her. You know, family or friends. Just someone who isn't wearing one of these." He touched the white coat in his lap.

"Wow," I nodded. "That's great."

Mark didn't look happy, though—no smile.

He gave a small shrug. "Well, it took me awhile, but I did track down a sister."

"Great."

He looked out the window at the darkening sky; the sun sets early in the late autumn.

"Yeah, well turns out the sister lives in Montreal. Used to live in a car but got some help and found a room. Yeah—a room. So she's poor, too."

"What did you do?"

"I tracked her down and called her to tell her that her sister's sick and that she should find a way to come here as soon as possible."

Mark traced the letters engraved into the plastic of his name tag, running his fingers over the black lines.

"Is she coming?"

"Yeah, at least I think she is. She said she'd take the bus down. Should be here by tomorrow."

Still no smile.

"So why aren't you happy?"

Mark straightened up, smoothed the white coat, and looked at me again.

"This morning I reported the news to my supervisor. I told him that I had tracked down the sister so that the patient won't have to die alone. I was proud of myself and thought he'd be happy, too."

"And? What did he say?"

"He wasn't happy with me, that's for sure. He told me that it isn't my job to hold hands with patients, and that if I wanted to do any more of that, I should go and be a social worker. Or a nurse."

"Damn," I thought, a familiar seed of disappointment beginning to take root.

"And he told me I'd lose my place in the program if I ever did that again."

And damn again.

"I can't afford to lose my spot," Mark went on. "I can't take that risk."

His hands lay flat and still on top of the white coat.

"Of course not," I answered. "Of course not. You shouldn't risk it."

The sound of traffic from outside seeped into the room, now full of shadows.

Mark stood up, shifting the white coat to the table beside him. I stood up and faced him—his green eyes were clear and direct.

"So, I've made a decision," he said. "I'm going to take off my values." He mimed taking off a coat. "And I'm going to pack them into a box." He acted out folding an imaginary coat and putting it into a box.

"And put that box up on a shelf for the duration of my training."

He reached up and placed the box on a high shelf, putting his values in storage. He brushed his hands together, in a "so that's that" gesture, and turned back to me. He half-smiled, and shrugged.

"I only hope they'll still be there when I can come back for them."

I nodded. "I have no doubt—absolutely no doubt."

Mark gathered up his things. I walked him to the door of my office and opened it onto the empty hallway. We shook hands and thanked one another. I watched him walk away. He paused at the heavy blue metal door and turned to offer a small wave goodbye. I waved in reply and went back inside my office, pulling the door closed behind me. I stood there for a couple of minutes, gathering the bits of my day, trying to stitch them together around the hole left behind by Mark's story. It felt like a battle on the verge of being lost.

~

When things slow with the coming of summer, the hospital staff members grab time for coffee and head outside for some air. The best seats are the ones under the trees.

This particular hot afternoon, a nurse I know well is sitting across from me, beaming from ear to ear, her coffee barely touched. She has worked at this hospital for decades. She's one of the pillars of the place.

She's been telling me a story of a new resident on her service—what a great guy he is, how stubbornly he stands up for what he knows is right.

"He says he knows you," she tells me.

"Yeah? What's his name?"

"Mark," she answers. "He's pretty great."

It's been three years since I've seen Mark—three years since I've given his box of values much thought. Time flows too full and too fast.

"He's like a dog with a bone," she continues. "I've seen him stand up for patients over and over again."

I think back to the woman in the ICU. I wonder if her sister ever arrived to be with her when she died. Three years ago.

"He saved a patient's life last week." The nurse goes on, "He pushed and pushed to be sure that a test was done when the senior guys thought it wasn't necessary. Saved the guy's life." She smiles again. "It really is great to see that in such a young doc."

I smile. "It certainly is." A streetcar rumbles past. "I never doubted that he'd be that good. Never once."

Battle won. Score one for the good guys.

Linda Clarke is a writer and storyteller and works with members of the health care community, including medical students, to help them see the power of story in how they understand themselves, patients, families, and other caregivers. In her years in health care, Linda has been part of many privileged encounters. One of them is the seed of this story.

WHEN THE WORLD
TURNS UPSIDE DOWN

A Doctor Experiences Being a Patient

I REMEMBER GOING TO A LECTURE IN EARLY JUNE, A COUPLE OF WEEKS BEFORE MY FAMILY PRACTICE RESIDENCY WAS TO END. I have always had excellent vision, and so, even though I had been up all night, I was surprised that I couldn't read the notes on the screen. "Something's not right," I thought. But my mind quickly talked itself out of worrying, talking back to itself with, "I must have strained my eyes from reading so much and working so hard."

A week later, I had to admit I couldn't read my patients' monitors, and so I made an appointment to get glasses. The eye doctor didn't ask me if I had any other troubling symptoms, probably presuming that because I am a doctor I would have checked out any other possible causes for my impaired vision.

In the next days and weeks, I also experienced weight loss, excessive thirst, and frequent urination. I remember drinking huge amounts of water and having to go to the bathroom between every patient. I noted that a pair of pants I had bought in May were falling off of me in June. Despite all of the clues, I avoided facing reality. Of course, if I had been one of my patients, I would have diagnosed myself in a minute.

At some point, the thought did cross my mind that perhaps I had diabetes. But then I argued to myself, "It can't possibly be true. I'm just worried and magnifying everything, just like I did all through med school, thinking I had every disease in the book."

My boyfriend, also a doctor, said, "If you're really worried, why don't you test yourself at work?" But I didn't. It was a good idea, of course, but somewhere in my head there was a voice saying, "I don't have time for this, and anyway, doctors aren't supposed to get sick!" Looking back, I can see that deep, deep down, I was afraid.

Instead of addressing my fears, I did what I usually do—I carried on. My residency ended in late June. As a treat to myself, I visited my grandmother in Florida for a week. While I was visiting her, I stood on some scales and discovered I had lost twelve pounds in two months. I decided I'd have to make an appointment with my clinic when I returned home.

At the doctor's office, I saw my physician's assistant. I must have glossed over or selectively shared some of what had been happening, because she didn't immediately say, "You have diabetes." Neither did she even do the obvious, like checking my blood or urine, which could have been done right there in the office. Instead, we started thinking about other things that might have caused some of my symptoms. Stress? Tuberculosis? A parasite?

I left the clinic having had blood drawn, which would be sent to a lab, and wearing a tuberculosis patch test. Both tests would give results in forty-eight hours. I went to my boyfriend's and just sat and sobbed. I knew something was terribly wrong.

I had been to the clinic on a Wednesday. By Friday, I was preparing to drive to Washington to write an all-day exam on Saturday. This exam was a big deal. You have to sign up for it a year in advance, the fee is about $1,000, and you have to pass it to be board certified as a family practice physician. Annette, a doctor and also a friend who would be writing the same exam, came over to my apartment. We were going to travel to

Washington together. I told her I had to call the clinic for some test results before we left.

I reached the office nurse and told her that the tuberculosis test was negative and asked her if the results were in from the blood lab. She started to read them to me. "Well, you're not anemic; your thyroid is fine; your blood sugar is 300. Wow! What did you eat?" I calmly said, "Oh, yeah! That's too high." And I hung up.

As a doctor, I understood that normal blood sugar levels are supposed to be between 70 and 120, and mine were 300. My mind was racing. All I could think was, "Can I pretend not to have this information until after the exam? How do I get myself to Washington?" Oddly enough, even though tears were streaming down my face, I actually felt a bit of relief. At least now I knew what I was dealing with. I quickly leapt into problem-solving mode.

I turned to Annette and blurted out, "I have diabetes! I know I have to deal with this, but I've got to keep going until tomorrow night."

Meanwhile, my physician's assistant was desperately trying to reach me, frantic that I'd been given my results over the phone. I was asked to come into the clinic right away. The standard procedure for a person newly diagnosed with Type 1 diabetes is to be admitted to the hospital for intravenous administration of fluids and insulin and for education. Quite predictably, I rejected that option, saying, "But I already know how to do all that stuff, and I've got to write an exam tomorrow!"

Even though I was emotionally seesawing—crying one minute and laughing the next—my attitude was, "Give me the fast course—let's get going!" On the checklist for stages of grief,

I'd already done denial and didn't have time for anger. I was negotiating and was ready for action.

My clinic agreed to try to work with my determination level. They set me up on an IV in a little office at the back of the clinic where I had access to a phone to be able to call family and friends. The nurse showed me how to measure and inject insulin and talked to me about my diet. In a matter of hours, I felt I had the tools I needed for the weekend. Annette and I were on the road, heading toward Washington. I was postponing dealing with the rest of my life until Monday.

Washington is my home, and so Annette and I had dinner with my parents. It was comforting to be there and to be able to talk things out. Even though Annette and I actually know quite a bit about diabetes, the scene after dinner looked like an elementary science class. Here were two doctors and my mother, a nurse, all trying to figure out how to read the numbers on a syringe and do an insulin injection. I caught myself thinking, "We are trained professionals who are supposed to know how to do this. I can't imagine how enormously difficult and stressful this must be for people who can't read or who are afraid of needles!"

I barely remember the exam. Getting meals and safely giving myself the appropriate amount of insulin consumed my mind. When I returned home after the weekend, I turned my house into "diabetes camp." Friends ate dinner with me every night, to be supportive and to learn my dietary changes with me. I read numerous books about diabetes. I went to the grocery store and read labels. I threw out "bad" stuff like six boxes of brown sugar I had in my cupboard and tried every kind of artificial sugar going. Most importantly, my blood sugar returned to normal.

When the World Turns Upside Down

I also took the time to see a doctor who specializes in diabetes. She was wonderful and somehow had the perfect balance of treating me with respect for my medical knowledge, but also being very clear that I was a patient. Because this was her field, she was able to share with me some of the hopeful developments in the world of diabetes.

"You'll be just fine," she reassured me, but she also said, in a very supportive way, "You don't have to do this all by yourself just because you are a doctor! In fact, I highly recommend you see a psychologist at least once. This is a really big thing in your life and it might help to have someone to talk to." She was right.

The psychologist helped me surface feelings of guilt I had about somehow personally causing this disease. The sessions also provided a forum for working through some decisions I've had to make in terms of my career.

Having diabetes has forced me to make sure my priorities are right. For example, even though I trained for three years to deliver babies and am good at it, I've chosen not to include that in my practice. Irregular sleeping and eating makes it much more difficult to control my blood sugar levels.

The last year and a half has been an amazing journey for me. I've had to make the transition from being a person with nothing wrong to a person with diabetes. In the process, I've learned that when you have a chronic illness like diabetes, you don't get to take a vacation from it. It's never going to go away, and it's hard work. In spite of being used to being in control of my world, I'm also learning that diabetes is a beast that you can't always control no matter how particular you are about management.

I've been so fortunate all my life. I've had lots of support and resources to pursue my dreams, and I've been good at what I've done. Now I'm trying to come to terms with things I can't do. Or, more accurately phrased, I'm trying to learn that just because I can do everything, I don't have to!

I'm slowly coming to accept that I'm a human being with some limitations. I've been criticized in the past for not taking very much time for myself. Now, I'm trying to do that and to feel comfortable with it. It's humbling!

It's also humbling to realize, until now, how little I really understood about people's daily lives. I used to think I was very aware of and sympathetic to the difficulties my patients faced. But now, I have a new awareness and new appreciation for the fact that lots of people are silently, privately dealing with a wide array of challenges. My level of understanding for how complex life can be, on a day-to-day basis, has become much deeper.

While I wouldn't wish a chronic disease on anyone, I am starting to see the positive impact diabetes has had on how I approach life and on how I approach being a doctor. I am gentler toward patients who have put off coming to see me, who have tried to pretend that whatever they have will go away. I also am more appreciative of the important, supportive, and useful role psychologists and counselors can play. Most profoundly, I think I now better understand the word "empathy."

———————————

This doctor went on to get a graduate degree in public health. She is now the lead physician in a community health center. She and her boyfriend referred to in this story got married and now have a young baby.

CREATING A CULTURE

I FIRST BECAME A PARENT IN THE LATE 1980s. Like so many first-time parents, I was highly motivated to be the best parent possible. I made it my business to read everything I could and become fully informed. I stayed away from microwaves, I watched what I ate, I was prepared to ask questions, to advocate for my children, and to protect them from harm. I felt empowered and resolute.

But all my best intentions and preparations mattered very little in 1991, when I learned that our new baby had a life-threatening chronic illness. Standing in a busy and crowded hallway of the Children's Hospital of Philadelphia (CHOP), my husband and I learned that our young son had cystic fibrosis (CF). As the doctor gave us the details about our son's illness, I remember wanting to find a place to sit down. My knees were buckling and I had to lean against the wall. As the doctor talked, I was distracted by a pay telephone that kept ringing down the hallway. I prayed that someone would just answer it so I could focus on what the doctor was saying.

As the doctor described the impact CF would have on our little boy, I saw my husband's eyes well with tears. I remember thinking, "We have been married for five years, and I have never seen him cry." I wanted so desperately to find a private place where we could be together and support one another. I knew it wasn't that this good doctor didn't know better or had simply neglected to find a private and comforting place to share this news. It was just that no physical space alternative existed.

From the early days of learning about CF, I felt isolated beyond words. I felt that no one, not even family and friends, knew what it was like to be me at that moment. Even when I was living at the hospital, with people all around me, I felt alone.

I sensed we were only seeing the tip of this iceberg we'd run into. I had no context in my personal life for living with chronic illness. I was used to solving problems, and I was desperately struggling with how I was going to fix this.

On our third night in the hospital, I was sitting beside our son's crib, still trying to comprehend what all this would mean for him and for our family. A nurse came in to the room and quietly said, "Mrs. Schlucter, a mom and her daughter were admitted last night. Her daughter has been living with CF for twelve years. If you want, I can introduce you."

Later that night, down the hall in the playroom, this other mom and I met. The nurse had ordered coffee for us. This mom was the first CF mom I had ever met, and she became my lifeline to the new world of cystic fibrosis. She had answers to so many questions that only another mom facing and living with the same news I had been given could answer. That nurse that night did something so small but so important. She honored the reality that families often need the unique kind of support that can only come from another parent.

I recall another small gesture from those early days. Our son's pulmonologist asked us if we would like to see what his team was looking at with respect to our son's lungs. "Come with me and I'll show you." It was such a privilege to walk beside this eminent physician as we traveled to the bowels of the hospital to the radiology viewing room. He understood that we wanted to know everything we could about our son's condition and that we wanted to be included in his care.

Creating A Culture

The actions of that nurse and that doctor stand out in my memory because, at that time, the Children's Hospital of Philadelphia had neither a culture nor an environment designed to support patients and families. Unknown to me at the time, CHOP was setting the foundation to transform itself from a world-class *medically*-centered hospital to a world-class *family*-centered hospital. I heard that the hospital was looking for input on what it could do to improve the experience of care, and so I wrote a letter to CHOP's Chief Executive Officer.

I simply described a day in the life of my family at the hospital. It wasn't all negative by a long shot, but I did describe what it was like to hear devastating news in a public place, what it felt like to have your sick baby as one of six patients in a room, and what it felt like to sit for prolonged periods of time in a busy waiting room when your child is ill. My basic point was to ask how such a world-class hospital, which provided such excellent medical diagnostic and treatment care, could be missing so many other pieces that make up the care experience for patients and families.

Within days, I received a call from the Senior Vice-President for Patient Care, who said she would like me to work with them to create change. The next thing I knew, I was sharing my story with an executive forum that included the Chief Executive Officer, the Chief Operating Officer, and the Senior Vice-President for Patient Care. As a group and as individuals, they were completely engaged. They connected emotionally. They were ready to respond and develop a blueprint for change.

Since that first meeting, I can say, unequivocally, that CHOP has totally and completely transformed itself and has exceeded every dream I had at the time. The hospital didn't just change programs—it changed its culture. It changed from a rushed, busy medical institution to a culture that now pays attention to the details of family-centered care.

This fundamental change was possible because both the hospital leadership and families were prepared to collaborate. Without the vision and commitment of senior leadership and their trust in the process of involving families, the sweeping changes in policy, programs, environment, and culture would not have been possible

In 1994, I had the honor of co-founding the family faculty program at CHOP. This program was designed to provide teaching forums for new employees, nurses, and medical students. I was one of five family leaders who were available to share our personal stories and experiences with hospital staff. We responded to invitations to speak, and we were happily overwhelmed by how many groups wanted us to speak to them, from biomedical engineering to trauma surgeons.

We discovered that these forums provided not just opportunities for us to tell our stories, but also safe circumstances for staff to ask the kinds of very basic questions they didn't feel comfortable asking at the bedside. For example, we were often asked, "Tell me what to say when I have to give bad news." I was so humbled by all of this.

In 1995, CHOP created the family consultant program, and I became the hospital's first paid professional family consultant. Today, this program has grown to having four paid professional family leaders on staff who meet with families, create programs, and bring a patient and family voice to communications and patient care.

Creating A Culture

Institutional changes continued. The year 1996 saw the establishment of the Family Advisory Council, which works to inform senior administrators, clinical leaders, and hospital committees at the strategic planning level. In 1997, a family resource center was opened that provides space for information, support, and other resources. In 1999, the Youth Advisory Council was formed. It recruits teenage patients who meet monthly to provide input to improve the hospital, socially and physically, for patients and families.

The changes at CHOP have been numerous. In addition to the innovations already mentioned, families are now given the choice to be present with their child throughout the care experience. Parents can sleep comfortably at their child's bedside, siblings can visit, parents make presentations at grand rounds, family consultants are part of the hospital's bioethics committee, and a parent co-chairs the hospital's task force on "The Ideal Hospital Experience." While so much has been improved, the hospital leadership believes that much more can still be done.

CHOP made family-centered care a priority. The hospital supported and sustained this commitment by integrating core concepts of collaboration, flexibility, support, and information for families into its programs and policies. The hospital is now nationally recognized for respecting and involving families as valued partners in the care of their children.

My greatest sorrow, to this day, is that I can't change that my child has cystic fibrosis. But my experience with the Children's Hospital of Philadelphia has shown me that I can contribute to other changes. I have also learned that when hospital leaders and families share a vision for what the care experience should be, and when there is an environment that supports collaboration, anything is possible.

Reflections

DIFFERENT STORIES, SIMILAR ECHOES
TO FIX, HELP, OR SERVE
WHEN ONE IS OVERWHELMED
THE INTENSITY OF MEMORIES
MOVING ON

DIFFERENT STORIES, SIMILAR ECHOES

SUCH DIVERSITY, YET SUCH SIMILARITY. In spite of the fact that each and every story in *Privileged Presence* is unique, what is striking is the use of similar phrases and the repeated references to what matters. In the straightforward reading of these different stories, whether from the point of view of a patient, family member, or health care professional, it becomes clear, over and over again, that it is the most simple things that make huge differences.

From Florida to Ontario and California to Nova Scotia, patients, family members, and health care professionals shared their unique health care stories. Yet, from this great range of geography, gender, age, circumstance, and perspective, what has emerged can be compared to the many different voices that make up a choir. Like repeating melodies in a major choral work, consistent themes about what makes health care experiences positive echo and resonate throughout *Privileged Presence*, creating a sense of harmony even though the notes are different.

The echoes from the patient and family sections of the choir are simple and include the following:

♦ Understand that first impressions are important and can set me on a path of fear or hope.

♦ Acknowledge me . . . say "hello"; introduce yourself; find out who I am as a person, and who we are as a family.

♦ Listen to me . . . I know what's normal and abnormal for me. I can help you figure out what's going on and what works and what doesn't work.

Reflections

♦ Honor my family as partners in my care, especially if I can't speak for myself. Please listen to my family. They know me well, can be my advocates, and can help you, too.

♦ Look at me, beyond my words . . . I may not say everything that I am feeling, but I may show you what's inside. My body language may help you read my heart.

♦ Share information with me and my family members, and be honest. Feeling ignorant and isolated is so much worse than knowing the truth.

♦ Appreciate any initiatives I may have taken to access information from sources like other patients and from the Internet.

♦ Take time to explain things and to ask if I/we have questions. If you help me/us understand and adjust, it will save time for all of us in the long run.

♦ See past what I have to who I am.

♦ Respect me for what I can do, not just for what is wrong with me.

♦ Ask me to consider treatment options and to be a partner in decision-making.

♦ Coordinate and communicate what you are doing with others who are involved in my care.

♦ Encourage me to participate, as much as I choose and can, in my care and treatment. I want to be more involved than simply following directions.

♦ Invite me to use my strengths and to participate in my care and recovery.

Reflections

♦ Consider what it will be like for me and my family when I go home. Help us plan, prepare, and know what to expect, and how to access help.

♦ Be flexible and bend or suspend rules when appropriate for my situation.

♦ Know that I enjoy knowing about you, too; it helps me feel connected to you as a partner in my care.

♦ Apologize. Say, "I'm sorry," and explain what happened if a mistake is made or if things don't go well.

These requests, or "invitations to provide good care," were cited directly or indirectly time and time again. Repeatedly, the stories in *Privileged Presence* show us how kindness, goodness, and common sense enrich health care relationships. They are simple acts of humanity and are neither complicated nor costly.

Many health care professionals intuitively understand how important it is to listen, to share information, to collaborate, to show respect, to take time, and to humbly pay attention. They know that the words they choose, the way they stand or sit, the interest they show, the gestures of kindness they offer, can make a difference to clinical outcomes and how patients and families manage their illnesses and feel about their care.

It is important to include these responsive elements of care in the training of future health care professionals. It is widely known that many medical students, for example, arrive with the values of compassion and collaboration, but that the older style of training extinguishes these values, rather than supporting and developing them. Think of the young man in the story "The White Coat." He needed positive role models rather than threats.

Reflections

The melodic notes that echo from the health care professional sections of the choir are well summed up in a quote of Mahatma Gandhi in which he was talking about "customers," but which is equally relevant to a patient or a family member:

> . . . the most important visitor on our premises. He may be dependent on us. We are also dependent on him. He is not an interruption of our work. He is the purpose of it. He is not an outsider to our business. He is part of it. We are not doing him a favor by serving him. He is doing us a favor by giving us the opportunity to do so.

TO FIX, HELP, OR SERVE

IT IS SIGNIFICANT THAT GANDHI USED THE VERB *SERVING*. In the world of health care, professionals spend years learning how to identify and *to fix* problems; their basic intention is *to help*. But there are profound differences between the verbs to *fix, help,* or *serve* from the patient's point of view.

Fixing stems from a judgment that the other person cannot do something, and the act of fixing takes away the potential for individuals to experience solving dilemmas for themselves. *Helping* usually occurs when someone stronger or smarter *assists,* which can result in the helper taking over and undermining the self-reliance of the person being helped. *Serving,* on the other hand, is the act of offering what is needed, what is appropriate, or what has been requested, without assuming that the person making the request is annoying, incapable, or powerless.

Serving keeps the focus of control more on the person being served than on the server. When you fix, you see someone as broken, and when you help, you see someone as weak. When you serve, though, you see someone as whole. Serving is more likely to create a relationship of equals rather than one of hierarchy.

WHEN ONE IS OVERWHELMED

ILL HEALTH AND INJURY CAN OVERWHELM EVEN THE SMARTEST, STRONGEST, AND MOST VOCAL AMONG US. Many patients and families who shared stories for this book were highly accomplished in their own day-to-day lives—business owners, elected politicians, lawyers, university professors. Some of them were even health care professionals.

And yet, many of them said they felt so completely vulnerable and intimidated by their health care encounters that they acted as though they had become paralyzed or mute. Comments like, "I didn't want to rock the boat," or, "I didn't want to make the staff angry" came from a sense of fear that they would be ignored or that care would be withheld. A comment like "I was too stunned to speak" was made when someone felt so disregarded that he or she almost felt invisible. How do you speak if you feel you are not even seen?

In some cases, people took evasive action and voted with their feet. It was as though it felt safer and simpler to change health care providers than to complain. But in some situations, the people telling their stories felt that there was no room for choice or change and that they just had to try to cope as best they could with the situation at hand. For example, the young man in "I'm the Full-Time Tenant of My Body" couldn't just get up and leave after his surgery when staff were not taking his complaints of pain seriously; he had to persist in trying to get the staff to listen to him.

One does not always have the energy required to challenge someone who has been inappropriate. The young woman in "The Journey of the Green Elephant," for example, was advised to reserve her energy for getting well when she was tempted to lodge a complaint about the plastic surgeon who refused to treat her.

And sometimes, it takes months or years to heal enough to truly find or reclaim one's voice or sense of self. Rachel Naomi Remen, in *Kitchen Table Wisdom*, says, "Somewhere along the way, our suffering subsides and our hearts begin to feel safe enough to open a little wider." The young mother in "Lingering Effects" took twelve years to open up again and honor her first pregnancy. The wife in "Flying Blind in a Frightening World" waited for two years before she gathered the emotional fortitude to confront her husband's doctor and explain what she had needed. And the woman in "A Profoundly Isolating Experience" surfaced from her ten-year journey and sent a letter to her husband's hospital six months after he died; in this case, it tragically fell on deaf ears.

THE INTENSITY OF MEMORIES

"What was the most touching moment during your time in the hospital?" provoked instant tears before the words could be formed.

"If you could say just one thing to a room full of medical and nursing students, what would you want to say?" stimulated a straightening of posture and lifting of a chin as the answer was spoken, with fierce conviction.

"What made your cancer treatment so positive?" evoked a smile of recollection.

No matter what questions were asked in the gathering of the stories for *Privileged Presence*, the answers were always clear and certain.

Health care experiences have an indelible quality. Whether a memory is fresh and new and only a week old, or is what one person called "twenty years mature," images, conversations (or lack thereof), small moments and gestures, and feelings of gratitude or frustration are imprinted on people's hearts and minds.

When our normal physical and mental functioning is uncertain, or when we are brought face to face with the fragility of life, all of our senses are heightened. As a result, health care experiences, for all the people who play a part in whatever the drama is, whether it be large or small, whether it be about birth or death, are situations that people remember with great intensity. How can it be anything but a privilege to be part of these moments?

MOVING ON

PEOPLE WHO OFFERED THEIR STORIES FOR THIS BOOK DID SO BECAUSE THEY SAW THE VALUE IN HAVING A COLLECTION OF PERSONAL REFLEC- TIONS ABOUT HEALTH CARE EXPERIENCES. They understood that stories could gently provoke readers to think about what makes health care experiences positive or negative.

They also liked the idea of the wonderful company they would be able to keep with others who were coming forward to be part of *Privileged Presence*. Many discovered a sense of their own wisdom and courage as they voiced their stories and said it felt good to share their memories. One particularly poignant interview led to an unanticipated but positive outcome of the storyteller realizing she needed counseling to process her experience.

The storytellers in *Privileged Presence* are not alone. The momentum for change in health care is building. The movement is toward a new system of care in which relationships and communication matter. Increasingly, patients, families, and health care providers are finding innovative ways of working collaboratively and compassionately, because they know they will achieve better clinical outcomes and improved cost-effectiveness.

It is comforting to know that so many people and organizations, in so many different ways, are working to improve the quality of health care experiences. Many of them are listed in the next chapter, "Building the Momentum for Change." Please get in touch with any and all of them. Find out what is happening, and offer your help and support.

"Never doubt that a small group of thoughtful, committed citizens can change the world; indeed, it is the only thing that ever has."

—Margaret Mead

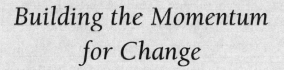

Building the Momentum
for Change

LEADING THE WAY:
KEY ORGANIZATIONS DEVOTED TO
IMPROVING CARE

- Institute for Family-Centered Care (IFCC)
- The Kenneth B. Schwartz Center
- Other Organizations Contributing
  to the Momentum for Change

~

USEFUL TOOLS FOR
PROMOTING CHANGE

- Patient- and Family-Centered Care:
  Definition and Core Concepts
- You Have the Right to Compassionate Health Care
- Partners in Care: Conversation Starters—
  A Tool to Facilitate Discussion
- Key Questions to Ask
- Educating Health Professionals: Approaches for
  Developing Patient- and Family-Centered Knowledge,
  Skills, and Attitudes
- Sharing Personal and Professional Stories

~

FURTHERING THE CASE FOR CHANGE:
SELECTED BIBLIOGRAPHY

LEADING THE WAY

Key Organizations Devoted to Improving Care

Institute for Family-Centered Care (IFCC)

FOUNDED IN 1992 AS A NONPROFIT ORGANIZATION IN BETHESDA, MARYLAND, the Institute for Family-Centered Care (IFCC) works to advance the understanding and practice of patient- and family-centered care in all settings where individuals and families receive health care and support. IFCC's twenty-four-member national advisory board includes patient and family leaders and representatives from hospitals, long-term care, public health, and medical and nursing schools.

Patient- and family-centered care redefines the relationships among patients, families, and health care professionals to create mutually beneficial partnerships. It encourages the sharing of information candidly and supportively. It fosters the active participation of patients and families in caregiving and decision making. With this approach to care, health care organizations and health care professionals invite patients and families to partner with them in quality improvement, patient safety efforts, facility design planning, and the selection and education of the next generation of health care professionals.

IFCC is nationally and internationally recognized for its leadership in partnering with patients and families, promoting change in health care organizations, and enhancing the quality of the health care experience. IFCC activities include:

♦ Convening annual in-depth seminars on pediatric, maternity, newborn intensive care, and adult health care for hospital interdisciplinary teams that include patient and family advisors.

♦ Sponsoring international conferences that solicit presentations and papers from patients, families, clinicians, administrative leaders, educators, and researchers from the United States, Canada, and many other countries.

♦ Developing and disseminating guidance publications, such as *Changing the Concept of Families as Visitors: Supporting Family Presence and Participation*; *Creating Patient and Faculty Programs*; and *Advancing the Practice of Patient and Family-Centered Care in Geriatrics*.

♦ Producing videos such as *Partnerships with Families in Newborn Intensive Care . . . Enhancing Quality and Safety* and *Patient and Family Resource Centers: A Visual Journey*.

♦ Publishing a newsletter entitled *Advances in Patient- and Family-Centered Care*.

♦ Providing on-site and off-site training and technical assistance to academic medical centers, community hospitals, agencies, and other health care organizations.

IFCC's web site serves as an important resource on the evidence base and supporting literature for patient- and family-centered care. In addition, the site provides profiles of individuals and institutions that have implemented patient- and family-centered care policies and practices. It also offers practical strategies and tools for how to advance this approach to care and how to create effective partnerships with patients and families to improve the quality of health care.

IFCC works collaboratively with many national organizations and agencies, including the American Hospital Association, the American Academy of Pediatrics, the Institute for Healthcare

Improvement, and the Vermont Oxford Network. Projects with these organizations have included a toolkit for hospital leaders, a policy statement and guidance publication for pediatricians, development of a innovative community to improve chronic illness care, and multisite national quality-improvement endeavors.

For further information about the resources and activities of IFCC, or about how to become involved, please visit: www.familycenteredcare.org.

The Kenneth B. Schwartz Center

Shortly before his death from lung cancer in September 1995, Kenneth B. Schwartz established a center dedicated to strengthening the relationship between patients and caregivers in the changing health care system. Ken viewed the Schwartz Center as a vehicle to advance the ideas, hopes, and concerns that he expressed in his article, "A Patient's Story," published in the July 16, 1995, *Boston Globe Magazine* (see the story "Making the Unbearable Bearable" on page 189).

The Kenneth B. Schwartz Center is a nonprofit organization with a mission to support and advance compassionate health care in which caregivers, patients, and their families relate to one another in a way that provides hope to the patient, support to caregivers, and sustenance to the healing process. The center's board of directors, initially composed of Ken's family, friends, and principal caregivers at Massachusetts General Hospital (MGH), has grown into a twenty-five-member board that includes professionals and experts in the health care, business, and nonprofit fields.

The Schwartz Center aims to strengthen the patient-caregiver relationship by:

◆ Promoting health care that values communication skills and interpersonal sensitivity.

◆ Offering unique forums for caregivers to give and receive support from one another.

◆ Increasing understanding of how patients define "empathetic care."

◆ Providing opportunities for patients and health care professionals to share their experiences within the health care system.

The Schwartz Center has developed and implemented the following programs:

◆ Schwartz Center Rounds—a multidisciplinary forum where caregivers discuss difficult emotional and social issues that arise in caring for patients.

◆ Clinical Pastoral Education (CPE) program for health care professionals—a program that gives physicians, nurses, social workers, and other clinicians the language, skills, and confidence to meet the deepest concerns and spiritual needs of patients and families.

◆ Grants—a program to fund projects that address core communication skills, particularly in the areas of end-of-life care, cultural competency, and spirituality.

◆ Compassionate Caregiver Award—presented to a caregiver who displays extraordinary compassion in caring for patients.

◆ Public education—an annual speaker series and panel discussions, open to the public, to raise awareness about the patient-caregiver relationship in our changing health care environment, as well as a newsletter and brochure entitled "You Have the Right to Compassionate Health Care."

For further information, please visit: www.theschwartzcenter.org.

Other Organizations Contributing to the Momentum for Change

Agency for Healthcare Research and Quality (AHRQ)
AHRQ funds, conducts, and disseminates research to improve the quality, safety, efficiency, and effectiveness of health care. The information gathered from this work and made available on the web site assists all key stakeholders—patients, families, clinicians, leaders, purchasers, and policymakers—make informed decisions about health care. www.ahrq.gov

American Hospital Association (AHA)
The AHA is the premier membership organization for U.S. hospitals and provides leadership and advocacy for member hospitals to improve care for patients and their families. The Institute for Family-Centered Care collaborated with AHA to develop the toolkit *Strategies for Leadership: Patient- and Family-Centered Care*, which is available for download at: www.aha.org

Center for Health Design
The Center for Health Design is a nonprofit research and advocacy organization of health care and design professionals who are leading the effort to improve health quality through architecture and design. www.healthdesign.org

Center for Medical Home Improvement
A "medical home" is a model for providing comprehensive primary care to children with special health care needs (CSHCN). The site has practical assessments and resources for providers in community practices and families serving on improvement teams. The complete *Medical Home Improvement Kit,* including measurements, strategies, and *A Guide for Parent and Practice "Partners" Working to Build Medical Homes for CSHCN,* can be downloaded from the site. www.medicalhomeimprovement.org

Clinical Governance Support Team
The National Health Service's Clinical Governance Support Team (CGST) is working with health care organizations in the United Kingdom to implement clinical governance as a systematic approach to assure the delivery of high-quality health care. CGST offers practical support through programs, information about clinical governance, and lessons from information related to this work. CGST is a co-sponsor of the Patients Accelerating Change Program with Picker Europe. For further information about activities that engage patients, caregivers (families), and the public in improving the experience of health care, visit the section of the web site that focuses on the patient experience. www.cgsupport.nhs.uk

Collaborative Family Healthcare Association
The mission of the CFHA is to develop a better health care model through the collaboration among family medicine practitioners, family therapists, and patients and their families. Educational resources, including selected articles from their journal, *Families, Systems, and Health,* are included on the web site. www.cfha.net

The Eden Alternative™

The Eden Alternative™ is changing the experience of aging and disability. It seeks to eliminate loneliness, helplessness, and boredom by promoting dynamic and humanistic environments supportive of caring relationships. www.edenalt.com

Emergency Nurses Association (ENA)

The ENA has been actively promoting family-centered emergency care. Their position statement, *Family Presence at the Bedside During Invasive Procedures or Resuscitation,* is available on the site www.ena.org

Improving Chronic Illness Care

As a national program of the Robert Wood Johnson Foundation, ICIC is dedicated to improving the experience of chronic illness care for patients and their families. This site provides resources about the Chronic Care Model, which views the patient as a partner with providers in decision making, participation in care, and quality improvement. www.improvingchroniccare.org

Institute for Healthcare Communication

Formerly the Bayer Institute for Health Care Communication, this organization has been providing education and resources to promote partnerships between patients and providers in clinical practice. The site offers many resources for professional development, including an *Annotated Bibliography for Clinician-Patient Communication to Enhance Health Outcomes,* as well as case studies and training resources. www.healthcarecomm.com

Institute for Healthcare Improvement (IHI)

IHI is a leader in advancing the improvement of health care. IHI's ever-expanding web site has a wealth of information on patient and family involvement in quality improvement and research, including strategies to capture the patient and family experience of care as well as to involve patients and families on evaluation teams. www.ihi.org

Institute of Medicine (IOM)

The IOM is affiliated with the National Academies of Science and serves as a nonprofit organization devoted to providing leadership on health care. IOM's major report, *Crossing the Quality Chasm: A New Health System for the 21st Century*, serves as a landmark publication in examining the problems of the current U.S. health care system and offering strategies for change. The report recommends that patient-centered care is essential to quality, safe health care and recommends collaboration with patients in clinical encounters and in the redesign of health care. www.iom.edu

Maternity Wise

Maternity Wise is a national program of the Maternity Center Association created to bring information and resources to support the practice of evidence-based maternity care to professionals, women, and their families. www.maternitywise.org

National Association of Emergency Medical Technicians (NAEMT)

NAEMT is an international membership organization representing emergency technicians, paramedics, and others working in emergency care. In 2000, NAEMT, in partnership with the Emergency Medical Services for Children, published a series of documents on family-centered emergency care that are available online. www.naemt.org

National Family Caregivers Association (NFCA)

NFCA serves as a clearinghouse of information and support for those caring for others who are aged, disabled, or chronically ill.

Leading the Way

There are a variety of stories and tools to empower family care-givers and promote advocacy. www.nfcacares.org

National Patient Safety Foundation (NPSF)
With its mission to improve the safety and welfare of patients in the health care system, NPSF provides resources, including a specific area devoted solely to resources for patients and families who wish to get involved in patient safety initiatives. www.npsf.org

Patient Decision Aids
This site is part of the Ottawa Health Research Institute and was created to assist clinicians and patients in working together to make difficult health care decisions. The program is research-based, and the site offers online tools, clinician training programs, and other resources. www.decisionaid.ohri.ca

Patient Safety and Quality Healthcare
This online journal offers numerous articles highlighting the role of patients and families in patient safety and identifying strategies and benefits. www.psqh.com

Patients Accelerating Change (PAC)
PAC is a program in the United Kingdom bringing patients together with clinicians and managers in hospitals and primary care settings to transform health care services. A resource packet with case studies and lessons learned through this collaborative work is available from the Picker Institute Europe and the National Health System's Clinical Governance Support Team. The web site includes a section on research about Patient and Public Involvement (PHI) in health care. www.pickereurope.org

Pioneer Network

The Pioneer Network is an organization bringing together elders, family members, administrators, nurses, physicians, other providers, advocates, and architects to promote culture change in all settings where elders live. www.pioneernetwork.net

Planetree

Planetree is a nonprofit membership organization based in Derby, Connecticut. It works with hospitals and health care organizations to develop and implement patient-centered care in healing environments. www.planetree.org

Professionals with Personal Experience in Chronic Care (PPECC)

This group of health care professionals established PPECC to advocate for improved systems of care after personal and family experiences with chronic illness and long-term care. Health care professionals are encouraged to share their personal experiences with the health care system in order to promote greatly needed change. www.ppecc.org

Remaking American Medicine

Remaking American Medicine is a PBS series that presents the current state of health care and strategies for improvement. The web site fosters the development of initiatives in local communities to improve the quality of health care.
www.ramcampaign.org

The Sorry Works! Coalition

This coalition, composed of all stakeholder groups, including health care providers, lawyers, and patients, is promoting a transparent model of disclosure of medical errors titled "Sorry Works!" Details about the model and related data are presented on the site. www.sorryworks.net

Voice for Patients
Voice for Patients is an organization devoted to empowering patients to be their own health care advocates in order to address patient safety concerns and medical errors. The organization advocates building partnerships between patients and providers and provides information. www.voice4patients.com

This list of organizations was prepared for *Privileged Presence* as it went to press. Because there is such momentum for change, new organizations are emerging to participate in efforts to improve the experience of care. The Institute for Family-Centered Care continually updates its web site as positive changes occur. Please visit: www.familycenteredcare.org.

USEFUL TOOLS FOR
PROMOTING CHANGE

Patient- and Family-Centered Care:
Definition and Core Concepts

Patient- and family-centered care offers a framework and strate-gies to address many of the themes and issues in the stories pre-sented in this book. By weaving the principles and practices of patient- and family-centered care into the infrastructure of every hospital, every emergency department, every office and clinic, and every medical and nursing school, the quality, safety, and experi-ence of care can be improved.

This definition and core concepts of patient- and family-centered care are presented as a resource for all those who would like to engage in improving health care.

Patient- and family-centered care is an approach to the planning, delivery, and evaluation of health care that is grounded in mutu-ally beneficial partnerships among health care providers, patients, and families. It redefines the relationships in health care.

Patient- and family-centered practitioners recognize the vital role that families play in ensuring the health and well-being of infants, children, adolescents, and family members of all ages. They acknowledge that emotional, social, and developmental support are integral components of health care. They promote the health and well-being of individuals and families and restore dignity and control to them.

Patient- and family-centered care is an approach to health care that shapes policies, programs, facility design, and day-to-day interactions of staff. It also leads to better health outcomes and wiser allocation of resources, and greater patient and family satisfaction.

The core concepts of patient- and family-centered care are:

♦ **Dignity and Respect.** Health care practitioners listen to and honor patient and family perspectives and choices. Patient and family knowledge, values, beliefs, and cultural backgrounds are incorporated into the planning and delivery of care.

♦ **Information Sharing.** Health care practitioners communicate and share complete and unbiased information with patients and families in ways that are affirming and useful. Patients and families receive timely, complete, and accurate information in order to effectively participate in care and decision-making.

♦ **Participation.** Patients and families are encouraged and supported in participating in care and decision-making at the level they choose.

♦ **Collaboration.** Patients, families, health care practitioners, and hospital leaders collaborate in policy and program development, implementation, and evaluation; in health care facility design; in professional education; and in the delivery of care.

Printed with permission from the Institute for Family-Centered Care.

You Have the Right to Compassionate Health Care

This tool outlines the attributes of compassionate caregivers and suggests ways for patients and families to participate in their own care.

Every patient has the right to compassionate care. Compassionate caregivers are sensitive and empathetic, demonstrating the following qualities:

♦ Respect for you and your family.

♦ Ability to understand your needs.

♦ Strong communication, listening, and interpersonal skills.

♦ Ability to impart strength and hope.

♦ Availability to you, especially in times of crisis.

♦ Ability to think and act creatively.

You will improve your chances for compassionate care if you view your relations with caregivers as a partnership in which you are an active participant. The responsibility for good communication falls both on you and your caregiver. Your role is to:

♦ Come to the visit prepared not only with your questions, but also willing to share your concerns. Your caregiver cannot read your mind, so be sure to express all your thoughts and worries.

♦ Tell your caregiver everything you know about your health and medical history, and what you think may have caused your problem.

♦ Take part in health care decisions. Address your concerns, both clinical and nonclinical (quality of life, work life, sex life) up front with as much detail as possible. Let the caregiver know what is important to you.

♦ Bring a friend or family member with you if you are worried you will not be understood or if you want support.

♦ Ask for a qualified language interpreter if you need one.

♦ Make sure the caregiver is talking in words you can understand, and ask for an explanation of any medical terms you do not understand.

♦ Tell your caregiver about all the health care professionals you are seeing, including alternative ones (e.g., chiropractors and acupuncturists), or any remedies traditional to your culture that you are taking.

♦ Show caregivers you are interested in them. Ask a question about how they are doing.

♦ Take notes and feel free to ask for written information. Repeat any suggested treatment plan, and feel free to ask the caregiver to write down his or her suggestions.

♦ Ask what you can expect regarding the treatment process (e.g., side effects) and the healing process.

The more open you are and the more you understand and participate in your own care, the more likely you are to receive compassionate care. If you feel you are not getting the compassionate care you deserve, talk to your caregiver. If the situation does not improve, look for another caregiver.

Printed with the permission of The Kenneth B. Schwartz Center.

Partners in Care: Conversation Starters—
A Tool to Facilitate Discussion

When patients are asked to evaluate their health care experiences, common themes consistently emerge. Over and over, patients and their families say they want seven key things. These statements are listed below. They all evoke the same obvious question: "Are we meeting the stated priorities of patients and families?"

Use these statements as conversation starters in a variety of settings, from professional staff meetings and health care training classes to quality-of-care committees and health care planning sessions. Turn them into questions and ask yourselves, "How are we doing? Can we improve?"

♦ Patients want to be consistently and respectfully involved in decisions about their health care. They want their families involved in ways they choose.

♦ Families want to be consistently and respectfully involved in decisions about the health care of their family member.

♦ Patients and families want health care providers to listen to their observations and incorporate their preferences about treatment into the hospital plan of care.

♦ Patients and families want and need useful and understandable information from health care providers.

♦ Patients and families want a personal connection—a relationship with health care providers. They need to be able to trust the people providing care.

Useful Tools for Promoting Change

♦ The patient's comfort and the control of his or her pain is important to the patient's perceptions of the hospital experience and to his or her family's perceptions as well.

♦ Patients and families want information and support for handling transitions in health care.

Printed with permission from the Institute for Family-Centered Care.

Key Questions to Ask

Asking questions is an exercise to reveal what it is like to be in someone else's shoes. Asking questions is often the first step to understanding how one's health care organization is experienced and perceived by others. Leaders of hospitals, clinics, and community-based organizations should ask the following questions about their organization as part of efforts to improve and ensure the quality of care:

♦ Do the health care organization's vision, mission, and philosophy of care statements reflect the principles of patient- and family-centered care?

♦ Has "quality health care" been defined, and does this definition include how patients and families will experience care?

♦ Does the facility and its signage create positive and welcoming impressions for patients and families?

♦ Are patients and families encouraged and supported to participate in care and decision making?

♦ Are policies, programs, and staff interactions consistent with the view that families are not "visitors," but instead allies for patient health, safety, and well-being?

♦ Are systems in place to ensure that patients and families have access to complete, unbiased, and useful information?

♦ Does the human resources system support and encourage the practice of patient- and family-centered care through initial interviews and orientation, as well as through ongoing education and evaluation practices?

♦ Do education programs prepare students and trainees for patient- and family-centered practice?

♦ Are patients and families involved in teaching students and trainees?

♦ Do patients and families serve as advisors to the hospital, clinic, or community-based practice?

♦ Do patients and families serve on key working committees, such as quality, safety, patient/family education, facility design planning?

Note: This tool can also be used by patients and families. They may wish to share these questions with their health care provider or with the leadership of the organization where they receive health care. This gesture might begin a dialogue about how to improve the experience of care in ways that are beneficial to patients and families, clinicians, and health care organizations.

Printed with permission from the Institute for Family-Centered Care.

Educating Health Professionals: Approaches for Developing Patient- and Family-Centered Knowledge, Skills, and Attitudes

The educational experience—undergraduate, graduate, and life-long learning opportunities—is critically important to shaping the practice and attitudes of health care professionals. This tool suggests content, teaching strategies, and support systems to integrate within curricula and the learning environment for students, trainees, and ongoing professional development programs.

In educational programs for physicians, nurses, social workers, and other health professionals:

♦ Provide opportunities to listen to the real-life stories of patients and families and to have candid dialogue with them about their health care experiences and the implications for professional practice.

♦ Include experiential programs in which students and professionals-in-training:

- Spend time with patients and families in nonclinical settings, such as visiting the home of a family caring for an individual with a chronic illness or life-threatening condition.
- Develop relationships with families served by hospital or clinic programs by working with the same families over time as part of assigned responsibilities.
- Attend a peer-support or family-to-family support group meeting that is facilitated by the participants.
- Work in a variety of community settings providing health, education, and support services to patients and families.

Useful Tools for Promoting Change

♦ Provide multiple and continuing opportunities for students and professionals in training to work collaboratively with patients and families and with professionals from other disciplines, such as:

- Attending a meeting of a hospital's patient and family advisory committee.
- Serving on a multidisciplinary design planning committee that has patients and families as members.
- Working on a task force with patients, families, and staff to develop patient/family educational materials.
- Participating on a hospital-wide patient- and family-centered care steering committee.
- Conducting and reviewing patient satisfaction surveys and conducting follow-up phone calls to participants.

♦ Integrate content on patient- and family-centered care when writing clinical textbooks and journal articles.

♦ Provide students and professionals in training with exemplary, patient- and family-centered health professionals from a variety of disciplines as role models and mentors.

♦ Provide opportunities for reflective practice that will enable students, trainees, and faculty to review and evaluate clinical, learning, and teaching experiences.

♦ Hire patients or other family members who have experienced hospital or clinic care as faculty and peer consultants for both clinical and academic programs.

♦ Model patient- and family-centered care, and involve patients and families in discussion and decision-making when conducting rounds.

♦ Require course work, reading, and discussion of patient and family narratives about the experience of care, the psychological ramifications of illness, and the importance of communication and collaboration.

♦ Honor the journey of becoming a caring, compassionate, and collaborative health care professional, and provide a variety of options for personal support for students and professionals in training (i.e., peer mentor, faculty mentor, access to professional counseling).

♦ Provide continuing education opportunities for faculty and other staff to learn patient- and family-centered principles and skills.

Printed with permission from the Institute for Family-Centered Care.

Sharing Personal and Professional Stories

Many people have an intuitive understanding of the core concepts of patient- and family-centered care but may not have applied them to their own health care experiences or their clinical practice. One way of opening this door to their own intuitive wisdom is through telling and listening to health care stories.

This exercise is designed to help participants develop an understanding of patient- and family-centered care by relating their own personal experiences to the core philosophical concepts (see below). This activity can work with any group but works best when the group is a mix of patients, families, and health care providers. It can also be used as part of the curriculum for students and trainees in the health professions.

Introduce the exercise: Explain that everyone is invited to think about and share a personal or professional story or experience that reflects patient- and family-centered care. Encourage people to share experiences that have created lasting impressions.

The stories should relate to the core concepts of patient- and family-centered care and can be positive or negative:

◆ Respect

◆ Strengths

◆ Choice

◆ Information

◆ Support

◆ Flexibility

♦ Collaboration

♦ Empowerment

Personal examples might include someone's experience with childbirth, being admitted through the emergency room unaccompanied by a family member, or the hospitalization or death of a loved one. Professional work examples might include how a physician's initial negative perception of a patient changed over time, or the way a nurse interacted with the brother of a young adult recently diagnosed with cancer.

Encourage everyone to share an experience, but be prepared that some people might not want to, given that this can be an emotional exercise. Offer to come back to them later or just let them "pass." They do not have to share a story if they are not comfortable doing so. Suggest that people be fairly brief — each person should take no more than two to three minutes to tell his or her story. You may have to be a gentle timekeeper.

If the group is large, you might want people to pair up and tell each other their stories and then, when the whole group convenes, ask for volunteers. This approach enables everyone to tell a story in a way that feels safe for those who may feel intimidated speaking in front of a large group.

During the exercise: Thank people for sharing as you go along. Occasionally link the stories back to the core concepts and point out how these stories help us see patient- and family-centered care from yet another perspective.

Conclusion: Ask participants what they learned from the exercise. Ask them how they might use what they learned in their exercise. Ask them how they might use what they learned in their lives or workplaces. Again, thank people for sharing their experiences. Let them know that stories touch people in long-lasting, significant ways. Encourage participants to use this exercise in other meetings related to patient- and family-centered care and for improving the quality of health care.

Printed with permission from the Institute for Family-Centered Care.

FURTHERING THE CASE FOR CHANGE

Selected Bibliography

This selected bibliography includes written and audiovisual materials related to patient- and family-centered care. For ease of finding materials related to specific areas of interest, they have been grouped under age-related and system-based headings: maternity care, pediatric care, adult health care, end-of-life care, patient safety, education of health professionals, and leadership and organizational change.

Maternity Care

Callister, L. C. (2004). Making meaning: Women's birth narratives. *Journal of Obstetric, Gynecologic, and Neonatal Nursing, 33*(4), 508-518.

Harrison, M. J., Kushner, K. E., Benzies, L., Rempel, G., & Kimak, C. (2003). Women's satisfaction with their involvement in health care decisions during a high-risk pregnancy. *Birth, 30*(2), 109-115.

Health Canada. (2000). *The Family-Centred Maternity and Newborn Care: National Guidelines, 4th Edition.* Available from Publications, Health Canada, Postal Locator 0900C2, Ottawa, Ontario K1A 0K9, (613) 954-5995 phone, (613) 941-5366 fax, and retrieved November 15, 2005 from http://www.phac-aspc.gc.ca/dca-dea/prenatal/fcmc1_e.html.

Hickox, Stuart. (April, 2002). Legacy of Angus. *Reader's Digest Canada Magazines Limited*, 171-198.

Maternity Center Association. (2004). Recommendations from listening to mothers: The first national U.S. survey of women's childbearing experiences. *Birth, 31*(1), 61-65.

Sweeney, M. M. (1997). The value of a family-centered approach in the NICU and PICU: One family's perspective. *Pediatric Nursing, 23*(1), 64-66.

Zwelling, E., & Phillips, C. R. (2001). Family-centered maternity care in the new millennium: Is it real or imagined? *Journal of Perinatology and Neonatology Nursing, 15*(3), 1-12.

Pediatric Care

Darch, J., Koller, D. F., & Patterson, S. (2004). When the going gets tough, the tough get playing: A child life response to the SARS crisis. *Child Life Focus, 6*(3).

Jeppson, E. S., & Thomas, J. (1995). *Essential allies: Families as advisors.* Bethesda, MD: Institute for Family-Centered Care.

Johnson, B. H. (2000). Family-centered care: Four decades of progress. *Families, Systems, and Health. 18*(2), 133-156.

Johnson, B. H. & Eichner, J. M. (2003). Family-centered care and the pediatrician's role. *Pediatrics, 112*(3), 691-696.

Koller, D. F., Nicholas, D. B., Goldie, R.S., Gearing, R., & Selkirk, E. (2006). When family-centered care is challenged by infectious disease: Pediatric health care delivery during the SARS outbreak. *Qualitative Health Research, 16*(1), 47-60.

McDougall, S., & Johnson, B. H. (2001). *Creating children's advisory councils.* Bethesda: Institute for Family-Centered Care.

National Association of Emergency Medical Technicians. (2000). *Family-centered pre-hospital care: partnering with families to improve care.* Retrieved on January 13, 2006 from www.ems-c.org/cfusion/PublicationDetail.cfm?id=000876

Society of Pediatric Nurses. (2003). *Family-centered care: Putting it into action, SPN/ANA Guide to Family-Centered Care.* Washington, DC: Society of Pediatric Nurses/American Nurses Association.

Tannen, N. (1996). *Families at the center of the development of a system of care.* Washington, DC: National

Technical Assistance Center for Children's Mental Health, Center for Child Health and Mental Health Policy, Georgetown University Child Development Center.

Thomas, J., & Jeppson, E. S. (1997). *Words of advice: A guidebook for families serving in advisory roles.* Bethesda, MD: Institute for Family-Centered Care.

Thomas, J., & Jeppson, E. (1997). *Words of advice: A training guide on families as advisors.* Bethesda, MD: Institute for Family-Centered Care.

Adult Health Care

Armstrong, L. & Jenkins, S. (2000). *It's not about the bike: My journey back to life.* New York: Berkeley Publishing Group.

Blaylock, B. L. & Johnson, B. H. (2002). *Advancing the practice of patient- and family-centered geriatric care.* Bethesda, MD: Institute for Family-Centered Care.

Feste, C. (1993). *The physician within: Finding motivation to combat a health challenge.* Minneapolis, MN: Chronimed Publishing.

Gerteis, M., Edgman-Levitan, S., Daley, J., & Delbanco, T. L. (Eds.) (1993). *Through the patient's eyes: Understanding and promoting patient-centered care.* San Francisco, CA: Jossey-Bass Publishers.

Glasgow, R. E., Davis, C. L., Funnell, M. M., & Beck, A. (2003). Implementing practical interventions to support chronic illness self-management. *Joint Commission Journal on Quality and Safety, 29*(11), 563-74.

Groopman, J. (2004). *The anatomy of hope: How people prevail in the face of illness.* New York, NY: Random House, Inc.

Groopman, J. (1997). *The measure of our days: A spiritual exploration of illness.* New York, NY: Penguin Putnam, Inc.

Hobbs, S. F. & Sodomka, P. F. (2000). Developing partnerships among patients, families, and staff at the Medical College of Georgia Hospital and Clinics. *Journal of Quality Improvement, (26)*5, 268-276.

Jadad, A. R., Rizo, C. A., & Enkin, M. W. (2003). I am a good patient, believe it or not. *British Medical Journal, 326,* 1293-1295.

Kabat-Zinn, J. (2005). *Coming to our senses: Healing ourselves and the world through mindfulness.* New York, NY: Hyperion.

Marks, R., Allegrante, J. P., & Lorig, K. (2005). A review and synthesis of research evidence for self-efficacy-enhancing interventions for reducing chronic disability: Implications for health education practice (part I). *Health Promotion Practice, 6*(1), 37-43.

Marks, R., Allegrante, J. P., & Lorig, K. (2005). A review and synthesis of research evidence for self-efficacy-enhancing interventions for reducing chronic disability: Implications for health education practice (part II). *Health Promotion Practice, 6*(2), 148-156.

McGreevey, M. (Ed.) (2006). *Patients as partners: How to involve patients and families in their own care.* Oakbrook, Ill.: Joint Commission Resources, Inc.

Moyers, B. (1993). *Healing and the mind.* New York: Doubleday.

Nuland , Sherwin B. (2005). *Maimonides (Jewish Encounters).* New York, NY: Schocken Books.

Payne, D. (August 22, 2005). I shouldn't have had to beg for a prognosis. *Newsweek,* 16-17.

Ponte P. R., Conlin G., Conway J. B., Grant S., Medeiros C., Nies J., Shulman L., Branowicki P., & Conley K. (2003, Feburary). Making patient-centered care come alive: Achieving full integration of the patient's perspective. *Journal of Nursing Administration,* 33(2), 82-90.

Remen, Rachel Naomi (1996). *Kitchen table wisdom: Stories that heal.* New York: Riverhead Books.

Sanghavi, D. M. (in press). Beyond the white coat and the johnny: What makes for a compassionate patient-caregiver relationship? *Joint Commission Journal on Quality and Patient Safety.*

Santorelli, S. (1999). *Heal thyself: Lessons on mindfulness in medicine.*New York, NY: Bell Tower.

Stein, M. (2003). *Mindful of the miracle: A memoir.* Toronto: Malcolm Lester.

Spero, D. (2002). *The art of getting well: A five-step plan for maximizing health when you have a chronic illness.* Alameda, CA: Hunter House Publishers.

Young, A., & Flower, L. (2002). Patients as partners, patients as problem-solvers. *Health Communication, 14*(1), 69-97.

End-of-Life Care

Block, S. D. & Billings, J. A. (2005). Learning from the dying, *The New England Journal of Medicine, 353*(13), 1313-1315.

Didion. J. (2005). *The year of magical thinking.* New York: Knopf Publishing Group.

Farber, S. J. Egnew, T. R. , Herman-Bertsch, J. L., Taylor, T. R., & Guildin, G. E. (2003). Issues in end-of-life care: Patient, caregiver, and clinician perspectives. *Journal of Palliative Medicine, 6*(1), 19-31.

Innovations in End-of-Life Care, an international journal of leaders in end-of-life care, published bimonthly (January 1999 through September 2003). While the journal will no longer post new issues, all 28 past issues are now archived and available at the following site: www2.edc.org/lastacts/

Public Affairs Television, Inc. Elizabeth Owen, Producer. (2000). On our own terms: Moyers on dying. (Available from New York: PBS Thirteen/WNET, 1-800-257-5126, www.pbs.org/wnet/onourown-terms/).

Sullivan, A M.,. Lakoma, M. J., Billings, A., Peters, A. S., Block, S., & PCEP Core Faculty (2005). Teaching and learning end-of-life care: Evaluation of a faculty development program in palliative care. Retrieved January 11, 2006, from www.hms.harvard.edu/cdi/pallcare/AcadMedJuly05.pdf.

Furthering the Case for Change

Patient Safety

Connor, M., Ponte, P. R., & Conway, J. (2002). Multidisciplinary approaches to reducing error and risk in a patient care setting. *Critical Care Nursing Clinics of North America, 14*(4), 359-367, viii.

Gibson, R., & Singh, J. P. (2003). *Wall of science: The untold story of the medical mistakes that kill and injure millions of Americans.* Washington, DC: LifeLine Press.

Gutkind, L. (Ed.) (2003). *Creative Nonfiction Issue 21, Rage and reconciliation: Inspiring a health care revolution.*

Entwistle, V. A., Mellow, M. M., & Brennan, T. A. (2005). Advising patients about patient safety: Current initiatives risk shifting responsibility. *Journal on Quality and Patient Safety, 31*(9), 483-494

Kenney, L. K., & van Pelt, R. A. (2005). To err is human; The need for trauma support is, too: A story of the power of patient/physician partnership after a sentinel event. *Patient Safety & Quality Healthcare, January/February*, 6, 8-9. Retrieved January 13, 2006, from www.psqh.com/janfeb05/consumers.html

Leape, L. L., & Berwick, D. M. (2005). Five years after *To Err Is Human*: What have we learned? *Journal of the American Medical Association, 293*, 2384-2390.

Education of Health Professionals

Blaylock, B. L. (Summer 2000). Patients and families as teachers: Inspiring an empathic connection. *Families, Systems, and Health. 18*(2), 161-175.

Blaylock, B. L., Ahmann, E., & Johnson, B. H. (2002). *Creating patient and family faculty programs.* Bethesda, MD: Institute for Family-Centered Care.

Greiner, A. C., & Knebel, E. (Eds.). (2003). *Health professions education: A bridge to quality.* Washington, DC: National Academies Press.

Ruder, D. B. (2006). Life lessons: Gravely ill patients teach medical students about listening and compassion. *Harvard Magazine, 108* (3) 44-51, 98-88.

Stewart, M. A., Brown, J. B., Weston, W. W., McWhinney, I. R., McWilliam, C. L., & Freeman, T. R. (1995). *Patient-centered medicine: Transforming the clinical method*. Thousand Oaks, CA: Sage Publications.

Leadership and Organizational Change

Advances in Patient- and Family-Centered Care (formerly *Advances in Family-Centered Care*), the newsletter of the Institute for Family-Centered Care.

Ahmann, E., Abraham, M. R. & Johnson, B. H. (2003). *Changing the Concept of Families as Visitors: Supporting Family Presence and Participation*. Bethesda, MD: Institute for Family-Centered Care.

Ahmann, E., Webster, P. D. & Johnson, B. H. (2000). *Creating and Expanding Patient and Family Resource Centers*. Bethesda, MD: Institute for Family-Centered Care.

American Hospital Association. (2005). 2006 *AHA McKesson Quest for Quality Prize Criteria*. Washington, DC: Author. Retrieved September 19, 2005 from www.aha.org/aha/awards-events/quest_for_quality/criteria.html.

American Hospital Association and the Institute for Family-Centered Care. (2004). *Patient- and Family-Centered Care Toolkit — Strategies for Leadership*. Washington, DC: Author. Retrieved September 19, 2005 from www.aha.org/aha/key_issues/patient_safety/resources/patientcenteredcare.html.

American Hospital Association and The Picker Institute. (1997). *Eye on the patients: A report of the American Hospital Association and the Picker Institute*. Washington, DC: Author. Retrieved on September 19, 2005 from ww.aha.org/aha/key_issues/patient_safety/resources/.

Boote, J., Telford, R., & Cooper, C. (2002). Consumer involvement in health research: A review and research agenda. *Health Policy, 61*(2), 213-236.

Davis, K., Schoen, C., Schoenbaum, S., Audet, A., Doty, M., Tenney, K. (2004). Mirror, mirror on the wall: Looking at the quality of American health care through the patient's lens. Retrieved November 14, 2005 from http://www.cmwf.org/usr_doc/davis_mirrormirror_683.pdf.

Frampton, S., Gilpin, L., & Charmel, P. (2003). *Putting patients first: Designing and practicing patient-centered care.* San Francisco: Jossey-Bass.

Hibbard, J. H. (2003). Engaging health care consumers to improve the quality of care. *Medical Care, 41*(1), 161-170.

Hibbard, J. H. (2004). Moving toward a more patient-centered health care delivery system. *Health Affairs, 0*(1331). Retrieved on September 20, 1995 from www.healthaff.org.

Institute of Medicine. (2001). *Crossing the quality chasm: A new health system for the 21st century.* Washington, DC: National Academy Press.

INDEX

Index

ABOUT THE AUTHORS

LIZ CROCKER's working career has included teaching, broadcasting, writing for newspapers and magazines, and running several businesses. She has owned and run a children's bookstore since 1978 and now has an environmental business with five stores across Canada. Liz has held leadership positions with a number of health care organizations, including the Izaak Walton Killam Hospital and the Canadian Institute of Child Health, and is Vice President of the Institute for Family-Centered Care.

BEV JOHNSON is President and Chief Executive Officer of the Institute for Family-Centered Care in Bethesda, Maryland. She is a nurse and has been a trustee of several organizations. She has provided on-site technical assistance and training to more than 200 hospitals and health systems in North America and has collaborated with the Institute for Healthcare Improvement, American Hospital Asociation, Association of American Medical Colleges, and many other organizations to advance the understanding and practice of patient and family centered care. She is the co-author of several books and the executive producer of award-winning films in the field.